AF797091

Praise for the *The Wise Woman's Almanac*

Connie Pshigoda offers wisdom, expertise, and guidance to every woman on their journey to wellness through all seasons of life. In *The Wise Woman's Almanac*, Connie has invested much time and energy to bring you a seasonal guide for physical, emotional, and spiritual wellbeing, from nature's perspective. She reminds her readers that God has given each woman an active part in their own health and wellness. Choices made can and will affect balance and harmony, as well as purpose in life. How she has woven nature's seasons with the earth's rhythms and cycles is brilliant! This book is a unique road map for intertwining health and spirituality that you will not want to miss.

—Judy Ponsford, BSN, RN, WHNP, and author of *You, God, Hormones and Health*

It's like a dear friend with wise advice. *The Wise Woman's Almanac* has become my go-to consultant for keeping myself healthy through the year. Each season, I like to review Connie's tips, especially the nutritional tips, for keeping my body and my mind healthy and nurtured.

—Michelle Poirier, author of *SugarLove: Broken Cookies Still Taste Good*

With God's wisdom, Connie has captured the importance of caring for our temple. In the Bible, 1 Corinthians 6:19 clearly tells us that we are the temple of the Holy Spirit. Connie causes the reader to understand it is a joy and a privilege to take care of our bodies. She helps us to see that eating in a more seasonal manner can benefit our lives and strengthen us so we can enjoy more of life!

Connie's practical approach to being wise about our food choices makes it possible for anyone to attain a lifestyle of wellness. I was intrigued in the first few pages by her story of growing up on a farm and how it prepared her for life. She writes like a friend who shares a lifetime of knowledge.

This almanac should be in every woman's home as a guide. We need to wisely take care of our temple, and thanks to Connie we have a plan that is already written out for us to follow.

—Gayla Bagwell, Editor-in-Chief and Publisher of SHINE Magazine

If you select food in a random or whimsical way, this book will open your eyes and guide you to new ways of choosing and preparing food that is in harmony with the seasons. *The Wise Woman's Almanac* is gracefully packed with wisdom and valuable advice. Your body and your health will thank you for integrating the lessons of this book into your life.

—Lisa Shultz, author of *Ready or Not, Tips for the New Grad* and more

The Wise Woman's Almanac

A Seasonal Guide with Recipes for New Beginnings that Never Go Out of Season

Connie Pshigoda

The Wise Woman's Almanac
A Seasonal Guide with Recipes for New Beginnings that Never Go Out of Season
by Connie Pshigoda

Copyright © 2016 Connie Pshigoda

All rights reserved. No part of this publication may be reproduced or transmitted in any form or by any means without written permission from Connie Pshigoda.
WellnessForAllSeasons.com

The information provided in this book is not intended to replace professional medical care or advice. The author and publisher do not assume responsibility for any medical action taken by the reader following the information in this book. The information is intended to educate, entertain and inspire the reader toward improved health. Some of the material within appeared in the original version of *The Wise Woman's Almanac.*

Scripture quotations, unless otherwise indicated, are taken from the Holy Bible, New International Version. Copyright © 1973, 1978, 1984 by International Bible Society. Used by permission of Zondervan Publishing House. All rights reserved. Other Scripture quotations are taken from the following: The Living Bible and are noted as TLB. Copyright © 1971 by Tyndale House Publishers. All rights reserved. The Message, Copyright © by Eugene H. Peterson, 1993, 1994, 1995. Used by permission of NavPress Publishing Group.

Published by
LCP
LenaClare Publishing
8200 S. Quebec St., Ste. A3736
Centennial, CO 80112

Books may be purchased in quantity by contacting the publisher directly.

ISBN: 978-0-9974170-0-5 (paper)
ISBN: 978-0-9974170-1-2 (Ebook)
LCCN: 2016904979

Cover and interior layout design: Nick Zelinger, NZGraphics.com
Book consultant: Judith Briles, TheBookShepherd.com

10 9 8 7 6 5 4 3 2 1

Cookbook | Health | Self-Help

Second Edition

Printed in the United States of America

To Jesus Christ, my Lord and Savior, my source in every season.

To my family, who has blessed me with four living generations of love, laughter and life lessons through countless seasons.

Contents

Recipe Contents

Nature's Late Summer Recipes: Indian Summer Delights

Nature's Fall/Autumn Recipes: A Hearty and Healthy Harvest

Nature's Winter Recipes: Tummy Warming for Bone-Chilling Days

FOREWORD

by Gladys Taylor McGarey, MD, MD (H),
internationally known as the Mother of Holistic Medicine;
Co-founder of the American Holistic Medical Association
and the Academy of Parapsychology and Medicine;
and author of *The Physician Within You, Born to Live,*
Living Medicine and *The World Needs Old Ladies*

How we live through what we are going through determines what we become. It depends on whether we make our decisions based on "Love and Faith" or "Doubt and Fear." This is a daily, hour by hour, minute by minute, living process.

When we become conscious of this truth and begin to take charge of our lives and destiny, books such as *The Wise Woman's Almanac* help guide our way.

There are many times in our lives when we may feel as though we have no control over what is happening. These times are very confusing and can be very frightening, but there are ways to learn how to move through these difficult times because we always have the ability to choose whether to be stuck or move, even by taking the next breath and being conscious of it. Once we realize how important and what a blessing this ability to choose is, we will find ourselves making the choice, even if it is to remain stuck.

Not long ago I had a patient in my office who was struggling with many problems—both physical and emotional. After she had spent a half hour telling me what was wrong with her life, I asked her to tell me what was right and good with her life. So burdened with the load of trouble she was carrying, she could not come up with one thing. I suggested that she take a deep breath and notice that she was alive and that was a good thing. I waited and she said, "I do have a home." Little by little she began to look for a few more things that were good with her life. Now she was beginning to look for the lighted path ahead and not the shadow of her past.

This was not a quick fix. She is still working and frequently finds herself dwelling on old painful memories which she has been unable to let go of, but she is on her way. She is not alone, we all have these times, but we also have Hope. When I was in medical school we were told, "Never give a patient false hope." I soon learned that that is wrong. I could not give patients false hope because hope is a spiritual gift; it is never false. Sometimes it is the only thing we can give one another. It helps to light our path. Every moment of our lives we have the gift of choosing whether we live in our own shadow or step on to our path forward with hope. As we work together, hope is the great gift we can share.

In the field of medicine, we physicians are asked to treat diseases, and we are taught how to do it. Our job is to diagnose diseases, and we are very good at it. However, if all we do is look for the disease and decide how we are going to treat it, we have lost sight of a very important fact: only patients can heal themselves. Our job is to use our skills and knowledge to support the patients as they do their own healing.

A surgeon can do a beautiful job of suturing up a laceration, but only the patient can heal the wound. If all I do is to look for what is wrong with my patient (make a diagnosis and treat the disease) and not what is right in their lives and how they can engage their life force, including their immune system, to do their own healing, I am not doing all I could do. We are all in this life together, and as we accept the reality and responsibility that our own life energy is doing the healing we need, we help each other. The physician within us and the physician without work together.

I recently heard a very touching news story about a young black man who had been in prison, on death row, for twelve years. Two years ago he was found not guilty and released. The commentator, who was doing the story, asked him if he was angry about what had happened to him.

His response was that he was so happy to be free and able to make choices for his life, he didn't have time or energy to spend on being angry. Hearing his story helped me, and I am sure it can help those who hear it with their heart. This is simple and so true. Why choose anger and pain over joy and love?

Often we are imprisoned, sometimes for years, in our own emotional prison. Yet if we took the time and energy to seek help and work with information such as *The Wise Woman's Almanac* brings to us, we could take the steps which could set us free. It isn't easy but, in the long run, it is a lot easier and healthier than being stuck and going no where. As long as we are alive, Life itself does the healing. Sometimes it does not take away the problem but gives us tools and the strength to deal with the problem so that we can rejoice in each sunrise and sunset we are blessed with.

So read and work with this wonderful book with your mind and heart open to choose your lighted path.

Gladys Taylor McGarey, MD, MD[H]

Section One

New Beginnings

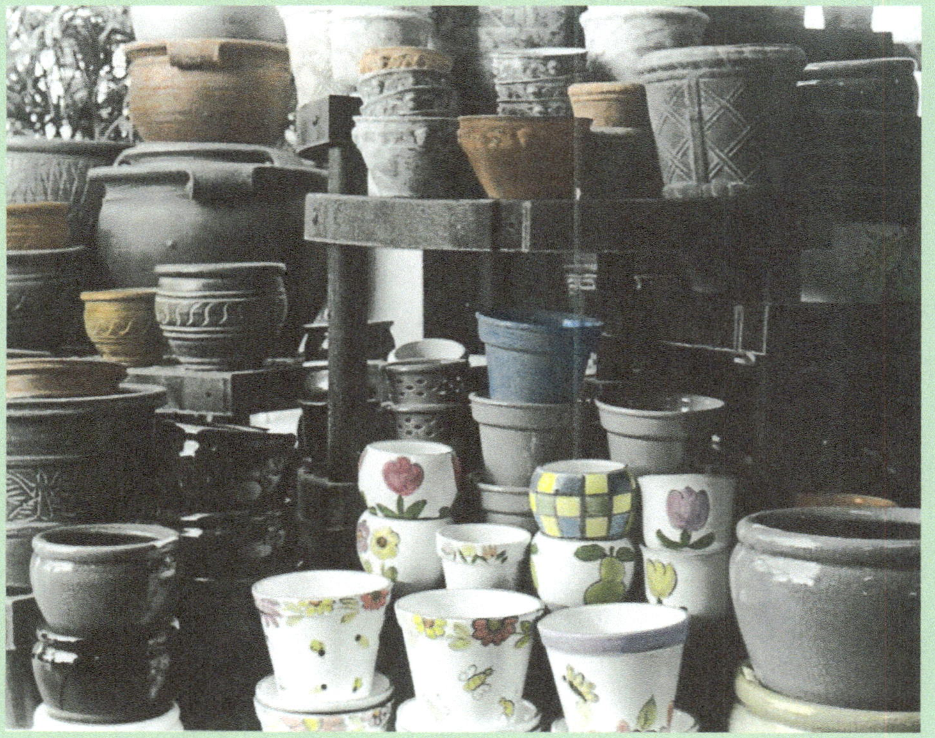

1

The Potting Shed: Getting Started

Dear friend, I pray that you may enjoy good health and that all may go well with you, even as your soul is getting along well.
—3 John 2

Remembering My Farming Roots

"Mom, I'm going outside to help Dad in the garden," I call as the screen door slams behind me. After Dad digs the last row, he waits for me to plant the seeds.

"There's my helper," he says as I run toward him. He hands me a bag of seeds and I carefully press them into the freshly turned soil.

I like the smell of newly dug, moist dirt. Seeing the sprouts peek through the rich soil and then flourish into healthy plants makes me feel happy and proud. I enjoy playing and working outdoors in God's nature. The farming and gardening chores sometimes seem endless, yet I accept them. I love the wide open spaces of my family's farm and take for granted the planting, harvest, rain and tornado seasons that come like clockwork every year.

As Dad and I hurry to finish planting the green beans, he points toward the sky and says, "We better hurry. There's a storm comin' up from the north." Spring storms in the Texas panhandle often bring rain, hail, and lots of wind, so I understand the urgency in his voice. I want my dad to know he can count on me.

"Let's get these tools put away or they'll blow into the next county in this storm," he shouts. I grab an armful of garden tools and empty seed bags as we both run to the shed to put them away.

"We made it," I gasp.

"Yep, now let's get to the house before the rain starts." He smiles and grabs my hand as we start running. While washing my hands, I smell supper cooking. Mom hands us fresh towels. "You two better be hungry because I've got a big supper for you."

The rain pounds against the window as we join hands in prayer around the supper table.

Valuing the Seasons

As a young girl, it felt good to be part of my farming family and the earth's processes. Sun, rain, wind, snow, falling leaves—I liked it all. During those childhood days on the farm, God planted within me a passion for the natural growth process. I appreciated the seasons, the soil, the planting, and the magnificent results. I still do. In those early years, I didn't realize how much the seasons would influence my adult life. Now that I'm a grown woman, having weathered many life seasons and several big storms, I value the lessons of Winter, Spring, Summer and Fall/Autumn. I deeply admire my hardworking parents and grandparents who displayed a generous love for the land and its Creator. And I now hold an even greater respect for the seasonal process.

The human body's physiological needs are profoundly influenced by the rhythms and cycles of the earth's seasonal changes.

Seasons change; we change. Over the years I have noticed similarities between the earth's seasons and the seasonal phases of our lives. I've researched, read and learned how everything in God's design—including the earth and his human creation—connects. The human body's physiological needs are profoundly influenced by the rhythms and cycles of the earth's seasonal changes.

When planting a seed into your garden or an idea into your life, the process transpires in much the same way. It takes planning, preparation, prayer and patience before tasting the fruits of your labor. Whether in farming *or* in cultivating health, relationships, solid finances, a career, or goals and dreams, it takes time to experience the reward. When you and I pause long enough to observe it, we notice the evidence of this cycle in most areas of our lives.

Whether in farming or in cultivating health, relationships, solid finances, a career, or goals and dreams, it takes time to experience the reward.

Your Journey to Wellness

The concept of wellness captivates my attention and curiosity and has for nearly fifty years. I define *wellness* not merely as the absence of disease, but as *the presence of physical, emotional and spiritual vitality and radiance.*

My God-given passion for the natural growth process logically evolved into my career purposes. I long to empower women to experience wellness throughout all their life seasons. My aspiration is to provide simple methods and practical tools for discovering and dispelling myths that many women unconsciously hold about their mind-body-spirit connection.

As I facilitate workshops and work with women one-on-one, many ask me to write down the nutritional information and methods I share. The book you hold in your hands is my loving attempt to share this valuable and exciting material with you.

Spring passes and one remembers one's innocence.
Summer passes and one remembers one's exuberance.
Autumn passes and one remembers one's reverence.
Winter passes and one remembers one's perseverance.
~Yoko Ono

This is not a "How to Be Healthy in Five Easy Steps" or "Ten Days to a New and Improved You" manual. My purpose for writing this book is to help you clear a path to better understand and fully experience each season as a new beginning. I've formatted this book to be a personal almanac for healthy living and well-being throughout the seasons of your everyday life. This personal guide will:

- Serve as an educational tool to increase your awareness and understanding of Nature's external seasonal influences on your physical and psychological health.
- Support you with a workbook and journal to keep personal notes and observations of your internal rhythms and cycles, your ups and downs, highs and lows. I hope you find this tracking tool helpful in increasing your understanding of your body, mind and spirit throughout each season—both environmentally and chronologically.
- Share several of my favorite seasonal recipes to hopefully inspire and encourage you to savor the flavors of each season in new and delicious ways.

Now Is the Time

Every enthusiastic gardener delights in her potting shed. I knew this even as a young girl. It's a place the gardener goes to enjoy and plan for the upcoming season. It's where she stores her tools, ready to be used for the next task or season. The potting shed provides a private space for remembering past gardens and dreaming of future gardens.

As you read and work through this information, I hope you will clear a place for your own potting shed so you may easily access your tools, chart each step of your growing process and plan your personal wellness garden. This place may be in your kitchen, your favorite reading chair or lawn chair, or perhaps a special place in your heart or mind. I invite you to jot down your vision for your personal wellness and get your tools in order. (You'll have the opportunity and space to do that in the next few chapters.)

Perhaps this seasonal wellness process seems a bit confusing to you right now. Relax. You'll soon understand how it works. Nature offers a simple approach to achieving optimum health. Please join me in a journey through life's cycles, making intentional changes toward fullness, wholeness and wellness. I'll be your guide in helping you plan and prepare wisely, nutritiously, joyously, and simply. Now is the time for this rewarding journey.

There is a time for everything, and a season for every activity under heaven.

~Ecclesiastes 3:1

2

Tools for the Task: Your Personal Almanac

He that would perfect his work must first sharpen his tools.
—3 Confucius

"BE SURE TO WASH those tools before you put them away," instructs Dad. "Don't put those tools in the shed with dirt on them. That makes them rust."

"Okay," I mumble, gathering the shovel, hoe and rake. "But this part isn't as much fun as planting." Obediently I place the tools on the grass. Then I hold the hose and watch as the cold clear water slowly dissolves the dirt clumps into the ground.

Designed for Purpose

Dad taught me to take care of our farm tools and equipment. He said each tool was designed to achieve a specific purpose. His "tender teaching" lessons have proved beneficial in many areas of my life.

Every diligent gardener realizes the valuable role tools provide in preparing, planting and harvesting the crop. Common tools in our garden included a shovel, hoe, rake, trowel, pruning shears, watering container, and a hat and gloves. I learned that we needed to keep each implement in consistently good condition in order to achieve our best gardening results.

You may own some tools for maintaining and repairing your home, yard, automobile, and computer but lack the necessary tools to support your well-being or repair degenerating health. Perhaps you have the tools for wellness, but haven't kept them in good condition. It's never too late to get your tools in order and redefine your vision of wellness so you can live with purpose.

Creating Your Personal Almanac

From the beginning of time the functions of the human body—or perhaps more accurately the "disfunctions"—have intrigued and perplexed mankind. Ancient physicians, healers and medicine men and women from every nation, tribe and culture carefully observed the body from birth to death. Those early observations laid the foundation for the modern knowledge and technology we appreciate today. For example, thousands of years ago, early followers of Chinese Medicine, Ayurvedic Medicine, Native American healing, and many other cultures, noted the close connection between nature's seasons and its affects on the human body, mind and spirit. These early practitioners believed that whole health was the result of living in harmony and balance with nature.

Contemporary research scientists remain both fascinated and puzzled with the functions and malfunctions of the human body. However, continuing discoveries and improved technologies help you understand more fully the simplicity and complexity of your design.

**As long as the earth endures, seed time and harvest,
cold and heat, summer and winter,
day and night will never cease.**

~Genesis 8:22

Your Journey to Wellness

Our original ancestors inherited dominion over that first garden called Eden. They accepted responsibility for the caretaking duties as well as their own selection of food and nourishment. Most of us in our current culture have wandered far from the simplicity and protection of that first garden experience. Instead, we gain much of our current knowledge about caring for our bodies and selecting healthy foods from sources that don't always place wellness as a priority.

It seems we've evolved into a convenience-first society. We often determine food choices by the ease or appearance of the packaging rather than nutritional value. This reality motivates me to share the wealth of information available on wholesome, holistic health and healing foods from Nature's pantry.

Previous civilizations recorded information about birth, sickness and death as well as external effects on the body such as climate, seasonal changes, food and water supply, and animal migration. These early almanacs chronicled annual data that often helped preserve entire communities. The information gathered from those early observations also helped people better understand who they were and how closely they were connected with their natural environment. By learning to live safely and strongly in each season, the ancient cultures left wellness wisdom to guide us in our modern age to achieve optimum health. I hope this personal almanac becomes a valuable tool in preserving and improving your health and well-being.

The methods I recommend and provide to guide you on your journey toward renewed health and well-being include the next five chapters:

The Feminine Route: Your Distinctive Map
Inner Conservation: Your Wellness Survey
Soil Preparation: Balancing Your Feminine Terrain
Internal Cultivation: Developing Healthy Habits
Landscape Décor: Adorning Your Unique Design

With each season Nature provides us the opportunity to participate in planting, growing, harvesting and storing, whether we are working with seeds for garden plants or ideas for the next great project. So, sharpen your shovel and let's dig in!

**Your mind is a garden, your thoughts are the seeds.
The harvest can be either flowers or weeds.**
~author unknown

3

The Feminine Route: Your Distinctive Map

You made all the delicate, inner parts of my body, and knit them together in my mother's womb. Thank you for making me so wonderfully complex! It is amazing to think about. Your workmanship is marvelous—and how well I know it.
—Psalms 139:13-14

I'M INTRIGUED WITH THE number of women I meet who are not familiar with their inner garden. Often they seem not to understand the purpose, function or location of their internal organs. And because they don't know the way their bodies work, they sometimes dismiss self-care as unimportant and then fail to experience optimum wellness.

Please take a few moments to study the illustration of the body's organs on the next page. I hope this visual aid will help you to understand your body more fully as you read through the information in this almanac. I really believe that with a broader awareness of your anatomical design, you can become more diligent and discerning in your personal health care and maintenance. You may want to mark this page and return to it for future reference.

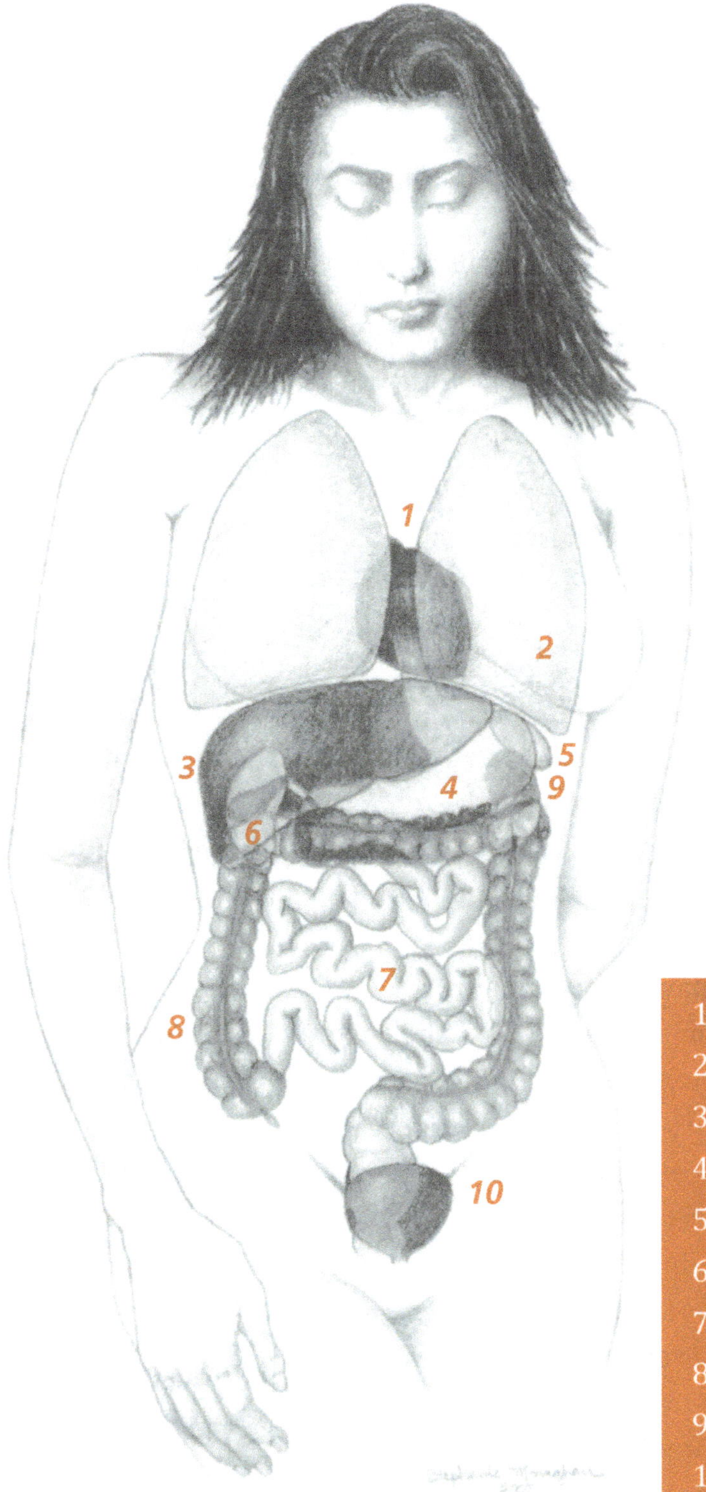

1 – Heart
2 – Lungs
3 – Liver
4 – Stomach
5 – Spleen
6 – Gallbladder
7 – Small Intestine
8 – Large Intestine
9 – Kidneys
10 – Bladder

4

Inner Conservation: Your Wellness Survey

Treat your body like a temple, not a woodshed.
The mind and body work together. Your body needs to be
a good support system for the mind and spirit.
—Jim Rohn, author

"WHY ARE THOSE MEN taking pictures?" I ask as Dad turns down the narrow road at the edge of the field.

"They're not taking pictures. They are surveying the land," he responds, driving closer to the crew. "They're using a surveyor's level to measure the contour and slope of the land."

"Why do they have to do that?" I ask.

"Well, heavy rains like we've been havin' wash out areas creating deep gullies that ruin the field. The surveyor's tool gives them the exact location of the field's boundaries and an accurate reading of the drainage slope, so I can prevent soil erosion and use the land more efficiently. It's all part of soil conservation."

Sometimes I didn't fully understand my dad's explanations, but I appreciated his knowledge and willingness to share with me, even though I was just a child. I remember how I loved riding in the pick-up with my dad when he went to check the fields. In those days, my dad drove a 1961 gray and white GMC pick-up that we called the Jimmy. Checking the fields meant anything from examining them after a rain or hail storm to analyzing the growth of the most recently planted crop.

Just as heavy rain storms and high winds can erode the soil in a poorly prepared field, unwise dietary and lifestyle choices can contribute to erosion of your health. To a great extent, your health and wellness rest in your hands. Wellness is an active process in which knowledge and awareness of body, mind and spirit health lead to wiser decision making, resulting in a higher quality living.

Age, ancestry, society, self-concept, spiritual beliefs, education, environment and economics greatly influence your choices, but don't totally define them. It's exciting to know that genetics determine only about thirty percent of a person's overall health and well-being. You have the privilege of considering who you are and what you wish to achieve as you design the remaining sixty-five to seventy percent of your wellness garden.

A tree with strong roots laughs at storms.
~Malay Proverb

Wellness Assessment: Getting to the Roots

As you complete the following statements and answer the questions, you'll gain accurate and specific information that will help you survey your total wellness.

Your Turn ...

1. My current health is: (a.) Excellent (b.) Good (c.) Fair (d.) Poor

2. I chose the above description because:

3. My desired health/wellness level or style is:

4. My past and current choices regarding my health are bringing me: (a.) Energy (b.) Joy (c.) Fatigue (d.) Sickness (e.) Other *(Choose all that apply. If you choose "other," explain what you mean.)*

5. What are changes I can make to achieve the optimal wellness I desire? *(List up to three changes.)*

6. I consider myself to be:
(a.) Energetic (b.) Sedentary (c.) Somewhere in between

7. How does my response to number six reflect or support my current lifestyle?

8. My sleep patterns are characterized by: (a.) Restfulness through the night (b.) Restlessness and interruptions during the night.

9. In the morning, I feel: (a.) Well rested (b.) Tired

10. My current sleep experiences affect my lifestyle in the following way:

11. When life stresses me to the limit, I choose to comfort myself by:

12: Afterward I feel:

13. I rate my self-esteem as: *(Circle a number along the continuum)*
    (Poor) 1 2 3 4 5 6 7 8 9 10 *(Strong & appropriate)*

14. For me, food represents:

15. I eat food when/because:

16. My childhood and/or teenage eating experiences have affected my adult eating choices or habits in these ways:

17. In what way/s do I eat differently when I am with others than when I am alone?

18. Some of my fun food choices include:

19. After I eat these foods, I feel: (a.) Guilty (b.) Guilt-free

20. I am a bedtime binger: (a.) Yes (b.) No

21. My favorite family food traditions include:

22. I was _____ years of age when I first became aware of my body image. The experience left me feeling:

23. The habits/patterns/choices/beliefs that encourage wellness in my life are:

24. The habits/patterns/choices/beliefs that limit wellness in my life are:

25. The wellness legacy I desire to leave for my children/grandchildren/other young women includes:

Only you can propose a health and wellness plan that works for you. There is no one-size-fits-all. You are beautifully and uniquely created so you will want a uniquely designed strategy for your own self-care. Nature doesn't stand still, and neither does a healthy body. For example, do you respond differently on a rainy day than a sunny one? Which do you prefer: a hot, cold, damp or dry climate? Are your responses different than the responses of your best friend or sister?

I suggest you spend a few moments each day observing how you feel early in the morning or later in the evening. Then while reading through this almanac, record and date your notes, responses and thoughts in your journal, so that you can check your progress and celebrate your successes. Many women tell me they enjoy watching for their own patterns, collecting information about what they need or want, comparing what works well for them, and then learning from their observations.

Eventually your observations will reveal how your personal rhythms relate to Nature's rhythms. As you collect this important information, you will have a full season of personal notes to guide you through future seasons. This will provide you with a powerful tool for healing and maintaining your health and well-being. Healthy roots produce healthy fruit.

Your Turn...

Review your response to the previous statements and questions and then complete the following:

26. A new discovery I've made about me is:

27. I'm beginning to recognize that every season brings change. Some changes I'm noticing about me are:

A Nutritional Survey: Your Personal Summary

Are you like many women today striving to balance a fast-paced lifestyle of full schedules, routines and responsibilities at work and at home? It's no wonder you may become disorganized, disturbed and dysfunctional. Sadly, if this disarray continues for prolonged periods, your body may experience discomfort or disease.

Just as the diligent gardener carefully notes plot size, soil type, drainage conditions and sun exposure in order to make improvements, so your notes and responses to the questions and exercises in this almanac can help you make positive changes in your inner garden. The following nutritional survey provides a tool to help you become aware of your dietary style so you can improve or improvise where needed.

Keeping a written record of daily choices or habits helps you easily observe what you already do that contributes to a healthy lifestyle as well as areas needing adjustment. You may find yourself in a rut, choosing quick, easy and familiar foods instead of fresh new foods that offer variety in color, fragrance, texture, taste and nutrient value.

Recently, a client sought my help with her health improvement project and was astonished with the information her written record of daily food servings revealed. Processed grains (breads, pastries, crackers, pasta and cookies) consumed more of her dietary intake than she realized. She quickly reduced the number of servings of those foods, replacing them with lower calorie, nutrient dense fresh food choices. Not only did she feel better, she lost some extra pounds. Now she does a quick nutritional survey quarterly to stay alert to her dietary habits.

You too can gain insight and learn to change your sometimes self-defeating habits. Now it's your turn to complete the following survey of your current dietary style. No one else is watching you write out your answers, so be honest with yourself. This is just another of the many tools designed to help you cultivate healthy habits and make wise choices for living well. You can do it!

When the diet is wrong, medicine is of no use.
When the diet is correct, medicine is of no need.
~Ancient Ayurvedic Proverb

Your Turn...

Complete the following thought-starters:

1. My typical breakfast may include:

2. My typical lunch consists of:

3. My typical dinner usually includes:

4. I drink ______ glasses of water each day.

5. My other beverage choices include:

6. My favorite snack foods include:

7. I snack ______ times each day.

8. My bowels eliminate ______ time/s each day.
   (a.) Easily (b.) With difficulty (c.) Painfully (d.) Other

9. Smoking does/doesn't *(Circle the appropriate word)* interfere with my desired wellness. How do I feel about the possibility of reducing or stopping my smoking habit or experience?

10. Excessive alcohol intake does/doesn't *(Circle the appropriate word)* interfere with my desired wellness. How do I feel about the possibility of limiting or stopping my drinking habit or experience?

11. I consume the following:
    1=never, 2=rarely, 3=often, 4=very often
    (Circle the response that most closely represents your situation.)

Fruit-fresh/frozen	1	2	3	4
Vegetables-fresh/frozen	1	2	3	4
Whole grains/nuts/seeds	1	2	3	4
Fresh fish	1	2	3	4
Chicken/turkey	1	2	3	4

Red meat	1	2	3	4
Pork/shell fish	1	2	3	4
Dairy products	1	2	3	4
Artificial sweetener	1	2	3	4
Condiments	1	2	3	4
Fried foods	1	2	3	4
Refined sugar/candy	1	2	3	4
White flour/baked goods	1	2	3	4
Pasta	1	2	3	4
Caffeine drinks	1	2	3	4
Alcohol	1	2	3	4
Salt	1	2	3	4

The human body continually works toward achieving a condition of health and wholeness. Old cells and tissues are replaced with newer, healthier, stronger cells and tissues. Your body receives and uses nutrients unique to your personal design. The choices you make today greatly influence your body tomorrow, next week and even next year. Maintaining your health is much easier than regaining it later.

Your Turn...

To assist you in maintaining your inner garden, please respond to the following thought-starters:

Good things that are growing in my garden of wellness are:

After completing the survey above, I noticed that I need help in the area of:

One simple wellness-focused step I will take is:

The information you have recorded in this survey will be a valuable tool as you prepare the soil of your inner garden. I suggest you date your responses and keep a copy close at hand to guide you in making wise and healthy choices for the next phase of the process.

5

Soil Preparation: Balancing Your Feminine Terrain

Mary, Mary, quite contrary, how does your garden grow?
—Mother Goose

"HEY, DAD, WHY DO you put that stuff on the field," I ask as he applies soil conditioners and fertilizer.

"The soil needs vitamins just like you do," he answers. "When several crops are grown in the same area, the soil nutrients get used up. Adding minerals and nutrients back into the soil keeps it well-balanced and ready to produce a high yield crop."

"Oh, I get it," I respond. *(But I don't think I really understood the process yet).*

Soil Samples

Later in my adult life and career I began to fully appreciate the importance of preparing the soil for a fruitful harvest—not just in the field or garden, but in the human body's internal terrain as well.
A well-seasoned gardener or farmer realizes the significance of testing the soil before planting. Proper soil preparation provides an environment for healthy seed germination and optimum crop growth. A soil sample test gives the actual condition of the soil at the root level of the plant. This test shows soil constitution, mineral content and balance and

pH balance. The gardener then knows how to supplement and condition the soil to achieve the desired crop yield.

The pH portion of the soil sample test is one of the most critical parts of the report. It shows whether the soil is excessively acid or alkaline, which determines the availability of nutrients for seed germination and growth. A favorable soil condition is essential for healthy, nutrient-rich, abundant produce. Much attention has been given to the over use of chemical additives that deplete the earth's natural vital nutrients, leaving it more susceptible to disease and pesky insects.

There is an important connection between the human body's inner eco-system and the earth's. It is essential to prepare your inner soil to produce and reap abundant health and harmony. Dr. Josh Axe, a Natural Medicine Doctor and Clinical Nutritionist, is one of many doctors who stress the importance of the body's pH because "a balanced pH protects us from the inside out." Do consider the importance of pH (potential of hydrogen) balance as a tool for cultivating wellness.

One cannot really understand the value of foods without first studying the soil, what it is, and how it contributes to life and health.

~Dr. Bernard Jensen and Mark Anderson,
Empty Harvest: Understanding the Link Between Our Food, Our Immunity and Our Planet

The Well-Balanced Body

You may be familiar with the pH balance of swimming pools or hot tubs and even shampoos and cosmetics for your hair and skin, but you may be confused about the pH balance requirements within your own body. The internal pH balance of the human body is extremely important to optimum health. Your body strives to stay in a state of equilibrium. Unfortunately, many modern day medical care providers overlook this valuable health tool. Examples of normal balance (homeostasis) in the body include:

- A normal body temperature of 98.6 degrees Fahrenheit
- Stable blood sugar levels
- Steady oxygen levels as well as carbon dioxide levels in the blood
- A healthy reading for bodily fluids that is slightly alkaline at 7.4

The human body is about 75 percent water. This important water supply provides the necessary system for a variety of substances (nutrients, wastes) to be transported where the body needs them. These water-based substances can be either acid or alkaline and are measured by pH.

When excessive amounts of the substances in the body are acid, acidosis occurs. Alkalosis occurs when more substances become alkaline. This pH imbalance in bodily fluids contributes to an increase or decrease in cellular activity which affects all body functions. To better understand pH activity, consider these points:

- The body's pH balance fluctuates with the changing seasons and conditions in your life. Internal and external variations challenge this delicate balance.
- The time of day you eat and how long it takes you to complete the meal affects your pH balance.
- Stress levels, sleep patterns, exercise routines, attitude and coping skills affect pH levels.
- Age, frequency of illness, medications and quality of supplementation play a role in healthy pH levels.
- Declining nutrient values in grown food due to industrial farming's overuse of chemical additives which deplete the soil.

When your body is healthy and fit, it can compensate for many challenges as long as they do not persist for a prolonged period. Listen to your body for clues of excess that may be leading to the following conditions:

- Excessive acidic conditions (pH below 7.0) may contribute to insomnia, water retention, frequent migraine headaches, blood sugar imbalances (type 2 diabetes), abnormally low blood pressure, acne, body odor or bad breath, frequent digestive complaints (acid reflux or indigestion), arthritic and rheumatic conditions, obesity, heart disease and a sensitivity to acidic foods (vinegar based, fermented foods or condiments).
- Excessive alkaline conditions of the body (pH above 7.4) may contribute to over-stimulation of the central nervous system, causing extreme nervousness or confusion, muscle aches, soreness and/or tingling, chronic fatigue or drowsiness, lowered immune function, digestive difficulties, dry, itchy skin, or leg cramping at night. Alkalosis is less common than acidosis. The healthy body is slightly alkaline.

When your body is healthy and fit, it can compensate for many challenges as long as they do not persist for a prolonged period of time.

Soil Preparation

Given the appropriate attention, pH balance can be restored and maintained. With a simple understanding of this acid/alkaline effect on your health, you can make wiser choices that will improve and support this balance. On your journey toward wellness and wholeness, you may want to test your internal soil by checking your saliva or urine pH.

Nitrazine (litmus) paper may be purchased from a health food store or pharmacy. These paper strips change color in the presence of acid or alkaline solutions. The scale is acidic from 0–7.0 and alkaline from 7.0–14, with water being neutral at 7.0. For best results, test first thing in the morning on an empty stomach. The healthy body's urine pH is slightly acidic in the morning (pH 6.5 – 7.0) and more alkaline by evening (pH 7.5 – 8.0). Follow the manufacturer's instructions and don't become stuck on exact numbers. You will want to follow this procedure for several consecutive days to get more accurate pH results. This tool can help you plant seeds for a healthier you.

Your body is in constant flow with its environment as your pH range will reflect. Remember that your amazing body displays several pH readings: your skin is slightly acidic (5.5) while your saliva is closer to normal (6.5-7.4) and healthy blood is slightly alkaline (7.35-7.45). Diet is the most influential and easiest area to change as you prepare your internal terrain. Your food choices on a daily basis will alter the pH levels of your blood, saliva, skin, and urine.

There are numerous charts, tables and lists available to introduce you to a beginner's basic knowledge of acid-forming or alkaline-forming foods. If most of your foods come from Nature's Pantry rather than the boxed, pre-packaged items on the grocer's shelves, you'll most likely maintain a healthy pH balance in your body. When you keep your focus on wise food choices, you'll be providing your body with the necessary ingredients to maintain pH balance with minimal metabolic adjustments.

Note the foods you eat most often. Observe any signs or symptoms you may be experiencing and simply start adding more of the foods that bring balance to your body while reducing the foods that contribute to the excessive condition.

Remember to include an adequate intake of purified water and to BREATHE. Deep breathing rids the body of acids and improves the pH balance. Mild to moderate daily exercise improves your breathing and oxygen intake. By replenishing your inner soil, you also improve the soil of your heart and soul. This is the groundwork in which creative ideas can be planted and come to fruition.

Your Turn...

To help you in assessing where you are right now and where you'd like to be, please complete the following thought-starters:

1. Foods I eat most often:

2. Foods I can reduce or eliminate from my diet include:

3. Foods I can add to my diet for a healthier pH balance include:

4. I usually cope with stress in: (a.) a calm, easy-going manner (b.) angry outbursts (c.) outwardly controlled and inwardly highly-stressed

5. I notice the food-mood connection when I eat these foods:

6. After an extremely stressful situation, I observe that my body feels:

7. I have noticed that my eating style changes with the four seasons in these ways:

8. My eating style has changed with my personal seasons (20s, 30s, 40s, 50s and on) in these ways:

Please date your observations or note your current season so that you can observe personal health patterns. Then you can make intentional decisions about how to optimize what you're already doing well and avoid what you're doing that hinders your health.

Balancing your inner terrain involves more than just ingesting supplements and watching your weight. It takes daily determination and dedication to cultivate healthy habits for a lifetime of overflowing wellness. Adding—*and using*—new self-care tools will help you become a more confident woman. And that is a significant part of living well.

6

Internal Cultivation: Developing Healthy Habits

Attention to the small gives character to the whole.
—Sarah Susanka, author

"GEE, DAD, I'M TIRED. Does farm work ever get done?" I ask as I help load the pick-up for a trip to the field.

"Not really," he replies. "Taking care of the land is an ongoing process, rain or shine."

We get some renewed energy when Mom cheerfully brings us a couple of lunch boxes and a large thermos of ice water. "Here you go, you'll want these if you're gonna' work in this heat," she says before heading back to the house.

Lessons from the Land

Once the land has been surveyed and restored, the conscientious farmer (like my dad) makes responsible choices in caring for the soil. Tasks that ensure a successful outcome include purposeful planting, irrigation, and soil maintenance. (Of course, Nature's timely contribution of plentiful sunshine, gentle rain and light breezes count as beautiful blessings by every gardener.) Nature teaches many lessons about caring for the earth, and much of that information applies to caring for your body.

Your simple daily choices affect your level of wellness, including the food you eat, the clothing you wear, the furnishings surrounding you, and the way you cope with life's inevitable stress. Just as it seems farm work is never done, caring for your health is an ongoing process. Learning to respect your body's natural rhythms in relation to Nature's external climate is an important action step that will help you achieve vibrant health for many years to come. Let's plow ahead.

Purposeful Planting

Like a prudent gardener who selects healthy seeds for planting and prepares the growing environment in order to produce a good crop, your daily decisions have a long term effect on your health. At the beginning of your inner gardening process, change only a few daily or weekly activities. Too many changes at one time may only increase your stress and frustration. Review your previous responses to the personal assessment and select a few healthy activities for your first steps toward inner gardening success. When these new steps become comfortable habits, choose two or three more new activities to replace the less healthy activities you are currently doing.

Activities or habits that you may want to plant into your new routine may include a monthly massage, facial or pedicure; eating less (or no) white sugar, white bread or processed food; drinking less caffeine or sodas and more water; or scheduling fun exercise or planned relaxation. A few simple additions and careful choices can produce many health benefits in your future.

Light is sweet, and it pleases the eyes to see the sun.
~Ecclesiastes 11:7

Your Turn...

List three new habits you want to cultivate this month:

1.

2.

3.

Solar Power for Living Well

The sun's rays activate chlorophyll (green pigment) in plant cells to produce organic substances (sugars) from carbon dioxide and water in a process known as photosynthesis. Similarly, sunlight provides numerous health benefits for the human body. Research findings tell us a few minutes spent in early morning sunlight leads to improved health, both physical and emotional. Disorders that have been improved with safe sun exposure include chronic skin conditions such as acne, eczema and psoriasis. In addition, Seasonal Affective Disorder and depression may be improved and the immune system strengthened when sunlight is present. Other health benefits may include strong bones and teeth, reduced risk of heart disease and lowered cholesterol and blood pressure levels.

Wise exposure to the sun's gentle rays lifts your spirit and improves your mood by increasing the production of serotonin, the "happy" hormone that promotes more focus and inner calm.

Today's indoor-oriented lifestyle often reduces exposure to healthy servings of Nature's light and this may contribute to a number of discomforts and disorders. Lack of sunlight may result in the following conditions: allergies, adrenal stress and insufficiency, auto-immune disorders, mood swings, PMS, obesity, and sleep disorders. Seasons and geographical locations are important factors to consider in determining sun exposure. The Winter season and geographic locations farther from the equator have reduced sunlight. Knowing this helps you determine the best time of day you can get your daily dose of sunshine.

Your Turn...

For increased understanding of your personal sunshine needs, please respond to the following:

My favorite sunshine season is:

I chose this season because:

Fresh Air: The Breath of Life

Fresh air and deep breathing promote a healthy body just as aeration provides a natural ecological balance in the earth's soil. Oxygen, the most vital element on earth, is our source of physical life. The human body can survive weeks without water and months without food, but only a few moments without oxygen. Your cells need oxygen to remain healthy and sustain life. Oxygen is a necessary element for all bodily functions. Most humans absorb insufficient amounts, which may contribute to fatigue, poor circulation, reduced mental acuity and brain function, respiratory weakness, or skin disorders.

The human body may also become oxygen deficient when fed devitalized, refined, processed, or synthetic foods. Heavy use of medications may contribute to toxic build-up and suppressed immune function, which also reduces oxygen efficiency. Chronic stress contributes to oxygen deficiency. It depletes vitamin and mineral absorption and produces stress related hormones. Breathing patterns affect oxygen intake and absorption. Insufficient aerobic exercise decreases oxygen levels in the entire body.

Sufficient oxygen promotes a stronger, healthier and more alive you. With this sense of well-being you are able to perform daily tasks and manage challenges with greater resilience and a sense of purpose. Have you ever watched a sleeping baby's rhythmic breathing—the deep-from-the-diaphragm gentle breathing? We seem to lose that natural practice as we take on the stresses of our adult life's season. Now is a good time to take a breather and listen to your breathing pattern. What do you hear? Is it shallow or deep? Quick or long? Do you become breathless after a simple activity?

Your Turn...

Respond to the following:

These are my observations after carefully listening to my breathing:

Now try the following exercise:

Sit quietly and comfortably with both feet on the floor and eyes closed. Breathe in slowly through your nose, expanding your abdomen. Hold this inflated position briefly, and then slowly breathe out through your nose, relaxing your abdomen, pressing the air out of your lungs. Practice this sequence until it becomes a comfortable rhythm. Try this exercise several times throughout the day to strengthen your respiratory system and to calm anxiety.

Water Wisdom

Gardeners know that watering is necessary to a successful harvest. No doubt about it, water is an essential element for healthy soil and the survival of vegetation. Likewise, your body demands water for healthful survival. The body is two-thirds water and needs adequate amounts of hydration in every season for optimum performance of digestion, absorption, elimination, circulation, lubrication, temperature control, and energy release.

The symptoms of dehydration often begin as subtle signs, yet they may lead to more serious disorders if not given proper attention. Insufficient water intake can lead to numerous adverse conditions including:

- heartburn
- back pain or general muscle discomfort and cramping
- migraine headaches
- colitis
- hypertension
- fatigue
- confusion
- constipation or reduced urine flow

Throughout its millions of natural metabolic processes, your body recycles countless ounces of water every twenty-four hours in order to maintain its normal physiological functions. Water makes up 83 percent of your body's blood; composes 75 percent of your brain; makes up 75 percent of the body's muscle mass; and accounts for 22 percent of bone structure. That's a lot of water and it needs to be replenished every day. Consider how these helpful tips can improve your water intake and usage:

- Drink water throughout the day—don't rely on thirst as an indicator.
- Drink a glass of water when you wake in the morning. This hydrates the body after a long period of sleep.
- Drink water before, during and after strenuous activity.
- Digestion needs hydration. Drink small amounts during your meal.
- Drink plenty of water if you have a tendency to be constipated.

Pure water is the world's first and foremost medicine.
~Slovakian Proverb

Conflicting beliefs continue on whether other fluids or beverages count as water intake. Many of the artificially flavored, colored and sweetened drinks or sodas actually alter your body's natural chemistry. The numerous sports drinks and energy beverages filling grocer's shelves should be considered carefully. Sports drinks provide different ingredients than energy beverages, which are usually high in caffeine, sugars or other stimulants that may over-stimulate the Central Nervous System. Please read the ingredient list and cautiously follow the intake allowance carefully. Pure, clean, clear water still takes the prize when it comes to irrigating your inner terrain for long lasting wellness and vitality.

Most proponents of a healthy lifestyle agree and recommend that drinking purified water daily improves most bodily functions. However, according to some experts in physiology and kinesiology, there is no scientific basis for the published suggestions for specific amounts of daily water intake. A diet plentiful in fresh fruits and vegetables promotes hydration. Herbal teas and freshly juiced fruits or vegetables also contribute to your body's hydration needs. If you don't like the plainness of water, try adding citrus slices or a fresh peppermint sprig for enhanced flavor and nutrient value. Still not sure about your hydration level? Check your urine: dark yellow and smelly urine indicates a need for more water. Pale and odorless urine means you are well-hydrated. If you don't urinate every two to four hours, you may be nearing the point of dehydration. Remember, your "normal" may not be another woman's normal, so note how you feel as you observe your body's rhythms.

When the well is dry, we learn the worth of water.
~Benjamin Franklin

Weeding and Waiting

The experienced farmer or gardener knows the importance of keeping the land clear of clutter. A neglected field can quickly become overgrown in weeds, creating smaller, less fruitful crops. If plants become spindly or puny, they need careful pruning for restored vitality. Weeding and pruning are important habits in cultivating an abundant crop. These habits also provide robust health.

A person's character and his/her garden both reflect the amount of weeding that was done during the growing season.
~unknown

Weeds know no season, either in your backyard garden or in your inner terrain. You must keep careful watch so the pesky weeds don't overtake your efforts toward wholesome living. When you weed out your unhealthy habits, you contribute to the improvement of your personal energy level, skin condition, mental alertness, sleep pattern, weight control and overall well-being.

Your Turn...

To help you take intentional action on your desire for increased well-being, please complete the following thought-starters:

I would like to experience improved health and wellness, so I want to remove the following weeds from my personal inner garden:

I will start doing this by________________[enter a date.]

I will ask________________________ [a supportive friend, colleague, family member, or coach] to help me stay accountable to my plan.

Pruning, the removing of unnecessary parts of a plant, is a vital part of the weeding process. Sometimes it may seem as though cutting away old, diseased or unnecessary leaves or branches will hurt the plant, yet the opposite is true. This healthy habit actually improves the growth and appearance of a plant. Likewise, it is to your benefit to prune the unnecessary or detrimental parts of your life.

Don't water your weeds.
~Ancient Proverb

Personal pruning begins with adjusting what you believe about your own health and welfare. You may believe some lies about yourself, your life, your health or your circumstances. Based on these lies, you might be reciting self-sabotaging statements everyday, either silently or aloud. Your self-talk—both positive and negative—indicates how you think and feel about yourself. These self-beliefs (whether they are misconceptions or the truth) can and often do show up in your body through signs of health or disease.

One of my clients came to me several years ago seeking my help in restoring her energy. After assessing her daily routine and health habits, I realized that much of her fatigue resulted from her self-talk. I listened as she told me that she hated to go to bed because she knew she would not sleep through the night causing her to feel tired and irritable the next morning. She repeatedly said how tired she was throughout the day and we discussed several steps she could take to change the way she thought and talked about her life. She agreed to speak energetically and optimistically about her daily activities and follow a set schedule for mealtime and bedtime until she experienced positive results. Within a few months, my client admitted she felt like a new woman. Her energy and vitality returned after she pruned the defeating self-talk and planted healthy thoughts and action steps into her daily routine.

So I urge you to cut out the negative, self-destructive or unhealthy statements you say or *think* about yourself, your abilities, your body or your appearance.

The way you think, the way you behave, the way you eat, can influence your life by 30 to 50 years.
~Deepak Chopra, self-help author

Internal Cleansing for Outer Radiance

Weeding and pruning are to the garden what cleansing and detoxifying are to your body. Your body's wonderful internal design allows for self-cleaning. Your body cleans itself with perspiration, tears, saliva, urination, menstruation, bowel elimination, and sinus drainage. The body knows when harmful organisms invade and is equipped to remove them. Our modern over-populated, over-polluted environment puts a strain on the body's ability to cleanse efficiently. You can help your body in this process. In addition to using the previous tools for wellness, you may choose to add an internal body cleanse.

There are many methods for cleansing and no one-size-fits-all. By researching and asking questions, you can develop a plan that works well for your personal style. Begin simply and remember to get your health provider's approval before you begin any internal cleansing program, especially if you have health challenges or are taking medications.

A one or two-day cleanse of vegetable juice, pureed vegetable soup or broth is the easiest and most non-invasive approach to internal cleansing. Eliminating solid foods and drinking vegetable juice or broth for a couple of days give the digestive and eliminative systems a rest without sacrificing necessary nutrients. Dr. John Douillard of the LifeSpa in Boulder, Colorado, warns against the extremes of many fad or trendy cleanses. Cleansing and detoxifying should be gentle and nutrient rich to avoid blood sugar crashes and cravings. Remember to always drink plenty of purified water during any cleanse. Perhaps you would like to try a simple cleanse for a day or two each month and note your response. When your daily diet consists primarily of real food, rather than factory formulated processed foods (high in hidden sugars and artificial ingredients), your toxic load will be lessened. Listen to your body. Let it guide you as to how long or how often to do an internal cleanse.

Skin Brushing for a Vibrant Glow

Another weeding-pruning tool for vibrant health is Dry Brushing—or Skin Brushing. Numerous cultures have used a variety of techniques dating back thousands of years. The Japanese used loofa sponges to exfoliate their skin prior to taking a hot bath. Following physical training, the ancient Greeks used a skin-scraping device called a strigil. Many Native American tribes used dried corncobs or sand from river bottoms for brushing their skin. Modern dry brushing tools include a long handled bath brush with natural bristles of vegetable fiber or boar hair. Avoid nylon or synthetic bristles as they tend to tear the skin.

Your skin is your body's largest organ with numerous functions beneficial to glowing health and is as important an organ as your kidneys, liver, heart, and lungs. You may be familiar with facial skin care and rejuvenation using cleansing, exfoliating and moisturizing but may not be aware of the health benefits of tending to the skin on your entire body. What's happening inside your body expresses itself through your skin, which is in a constant state of renewal. Skin brushing (or dry brushing) assists in stabilizing the normal functions of your skin by exfoliating dead skin cells from the outer surface, stimulating lymphatic drainage of the skin, increasing venous blood flow, and toning and activating muscles and nerves. Skin brushing brings a youthful glow to neglected or mistreated skin. I suggest you begin your skin brushing ritual with these steps:

- Find *your* best time to dry brush. Perhaps it will be when you awake in the morning, or after an exercise workout or massage, before a shower, bath or bedtime.
- With the dry brush on dry skin and using firm but not heavy pressure, begin brushing about four to five strokes on legs and arms (from toes or fingers UP toward the heart). Use circular strokes in the armpits and on your buttocks. Brush the top and bottom of your feet to stimulate the reflex points. Increase to six to seven strokes as your skin becomes seasoned.
- Do not brush your face, breasts, any open sores or active metastatic cancer condition.

Adequate nourishment of the cells and sufficient oxygenation are not possible when waste and toxins are present. Cells that are not nourished sufficiently can cause premature aging and illness.
~Mildred Carter and Tammy Weber,
Body Reflexology, Healing at Your Fingertips

Necessary Rest: Fallow Ground and Crop Rotation

Experienced farmers and gardeners know the importance of resting the soil and rotating the crops in order to take care of the land and produce consistently abundant harvests. Depending on the geographical area and its conditions, farmers learn to cultivate different crops during different seasons and climates.

A field or garden plot left unplanted or inactive (fallow) for a season uses this resting time to rebuild its nutrient supply. Rest is also important to *your* wellness. A tired body becomes a sick body.

Your Turn...

For increased personal awareness, respond to the following:

When was the last time I felt *really* rested?

What did I do to feel that way?

How often do I allow myself to truly rest?

Some restful experiences that I enjoy most (or desire to enjoy) include:

The wise farmer plans ahead for the crop planting and resting cycles in order to get the most from the earth and its rich supplies. Likewise, your health will blossom when you intentionally plan your resting times and activity times.

Take a rest: a field that has rested gives a bountiful crop.
~Ovid, first century Roman poet

Recent newspaper headlines, magazine articles, television and radio advertisements alert us to the adverse effects of the sleep-deprived brain. Most Americans do not get enough sleep. Research clearly indicates that a full night (seven to eight hours) of sound sleep reduces stress, aging, obesity, and improves your immune system, brain function and overall daily performance. The American Academy of Sleep Medicine provides education and research in the study of sleep disorders and solutions. This may be a good source to contact if disruptive sleep patterns negatively affect your daily routine.

There may be many reasons for poor sleeping patterns and if you're having trouble sleeping, you may benefit from professional medical care. To help you and your doctor or health consultant, you may wish to keep a sleep journal. This practice often helps uncover possible behaviors or circumstances that interfere with your restful sleep. Each morning when you awake, briefly note your sleep pattern from the previous night in a notebook or your sleep journal. In time, you may discover patterns or cycles emerging that can offer helpful insight and assist you in finding methods for improvement.

The human body has adapted to its current artificial surroundings (lighting, sounds, fragrances) away from its natural biological clock which drives its circadian rhythm. We no longer arise and retire with the sun's cycle. If we cannot spend time outdoors, there are special lights to imitate the sun. The sounds of nature can now be heard digitally. The glow from our electronic devices passes through our eye's retina into the part of our brain (hypothalamus) that controls our body's sleep activity, slowing the release of melatonin, the sleep-inducing hormone. A good rest is more than a beauty aid—it's life enhancing.

The following beneficial habits may bring about restful, health-giving sleep. You may wish to revise your bedtime ritual to include calming activities such as:

- Taking a relaxing bath with Epsom Salts or essential oils
- Listening to peaceful music to help slow down cognitive stimulation
- Reading an inspirational book or magazine—*not* on your digital device
- Sipping a cup of chamomile tea and giving yourself permission to rest
- Unplugging and powering down from your computer, television or phone

And God blessed the seventh day and made it holy, because on it he rested from all the work of creating that he had done.
~Genesis 2:3

Change Is Good for Your Health

Crop rotation is another method used by the dedicated farmer and gardener to promote plentiful crops and provide for the land. By planting a different crop each season, the farmer protects the soil's nutrient supply and maintains the integrity of the soil. Similarly, by rotating and varying your personal diet and activities, you can protect, maintain and enhance your health and wellness. An "in-season" meal prepared with a variety of color, texture, flavor and aroma can provide complete nutrient value and dining pleasure.

Today's hurried lifestyle leads many women into a routine rut that depletes their energy and enthusiasm for life as well as their vital nutrients. You may wish to vary your exercise program with the seasons to prevent boredom and burnout. This is a great way to appreciate the gifts each change of season offers. You can learn to balance your work time with play or rest time.

For women constantly on the go, I often recommend a brief *silence sabbatical*. With so much noise pollution from cell phones, computers, traffic, office chatter, buzzers, bells and beepers, your mind needs a rest. Indulge yourself a few minutes each day in complete silence.

Your Turn...

Please take a few moments to respond to the following:

What are some ways I can rotate my activities to bring my routine into healthier balance?

What do I hear when everything is silent?

When I listen to my body, what does it tell me it needs?

Soulful Gardening

Have you ever pondered the overall health benefits of cultivating fairness, generosity, curiosity, patience, hospitality, courage or respect? I once heard an old saying that "the depth of our being is often unknown until we are uprooted." I believe that nurturing these virtues may help you to stay well-grounded during life's storms. Just as we desire a bumper crop in our outdoor garden, tending to our spiritual fruit also contributes to our overall wholesomeness. Galatians 5:22 in the New Testament teaches that the fruit of the Spirit includes love, joy, peace, patience, kindness, goodness, faithfulness, gentleness, and self-control. A verbal attack, rejection or betrayal may still leave a sting, but you'll find yourself on solid ground when your emotional tap root is strongly attached to healthy knowledge, beliefs and habits. When you've been a good steward physically, mentally, emotionally, and spiritually, these unexpected storms will not completely destroy your inner garden. The following 5-R's to Renewal seem to sum up the steps you can take to cultivate healthy habits and grow yourself into the wise woman you desire to be.

Prepare a fallow heart to welcome mystery,
water a dormant soul with springs of joy.
Cultivate awe. Plant a seed of hope.
~Joyce Hollyday, Minister

The 5-R's to Renewal

1. **Remove:** Discontinue any *unhealthy* habits you've developed or *destructive* lifestyle choices you've made concerning your diet, sleep, activities, attitude, posture, water in-take, exercise, relationships or a hopeless (or helpless) life outlook.

2. **Replace:** To achieve the *healthy* lifestyle you desire, create a new plan relating to your diet, sleep habits, exercise, spirituality, recreation, emotions and relationships. You can replace your self-defeating patterns with an optimistic and relaxed attitude, a strong faith, a wise diet and an enjoyable exercise routine. With determination, God's help, and others' support, you can do it. You will then move past obstacles and become the woman you dream of being.

3. **Rebalance:** Coordinate your new healthy choices into an ongoing strategic plan that works well for *you*. Be gentle with yourself. Try not to add to your stress level by comparing yourself to someone else and her wellness plan. By taking small steps in the beginning and adding new steps as you progress, you will achieve your goals. Focus on personal goals, home goals and career goals in phases. Give yourself a break and adapt gradually to your new wellness style.

4. **Repair/Restore:** Organ function and cellular activity show improvement as you cultivate new healthy habits. The small steps you take in these areas will bring healing to your *roots.* Be encouraged. Eventually, you will see and feel physical and emotional vitality. Stay with the process and be patient.

5. **Rejoice:** Develop a joy-filled, glad and grateful heart. Take time each day (and each season) to appreciate *and celebrate* the good things in your life, the wise choices you are making, and your forward movement toward wellness. Perhaps you'd like to create a Gratitude Journal. Several times each week, perhaps in the morning before you start your day or in the evening before you retire, you can jot down the ways you are thankful. Allow yourself to love, laugh and live each day to your fullest capacity.

But I will restore you to health and heal your wounds, declares the LORD.
~Jeremiah 30:17

Perhaps this all seems a little (or a lot) overwhelming right now. I assure you that it is a step-by-step process and cannot be accomplished overnight, in one week or even in one month. These wise life changes will take time to become new healthy habits, and that's okay, so get started. It takes just one small choice at a time, one moment at a time.

Your Turn...

My "in the moment" challenge to you is to respond to the following question before *reading on. Write your response below and then share it with a friend.*

What one new action step will I take this week—starting tomorrow?

Going the Distance

As a young girl on our farm, I wanted quick results, yet I learned the value of cultivating for the long haul. My youthful impatience gave way to excitement once harvest season arrived. It is my desire that each of you stay the course, practice patience and intentionality, and then reap the benefits of optimum health. I hope you're in it for the long haul. In the meantime, if the journey gets boring, may you find delight in decorating your garden path but keep moving ahead.

I can hardly wait for tomorrow, it means a new life for me each and every day.
~Stanley Kunitz, 1905-2006, American poet

7

Landscape Décor: Adorning Your Unique Design

Beauty is how you feel inside, and it reflects in your eyes. It is not something physical.
—Sophia Loren, actress

"WHERE DO YOU WANT me to put this?" I call, as I lug a rusty old cream can from the Quonset to our garden.

"Just put it here," Mom answers and points to a place near the gate. I love family work days—and it isn't even Saturday.

"Look what I found," my sister shrieks, holding up several tarnished and bent spoons and forks.

"Oh, those were your grandma's," says my dad. "I think we can use 'em to make wind chimes to hang in the fruit tree. That might scare a bird or two away from the mulberries!"

The buildings on our farm included a livestock barn, chicken house, Quonset (a half cylinder shaped metal building where we stored farm equipment), granary and garage. Each building bulged with an accumulation of left-behind and worn-out tools, appliances, furniture, toys and assorted odds and ends. My grandparents lived on and farmed the land before we moved there, and they left many memories of their lives behind. Their leftovers became my treasures.

We decorated our yard and garden with iron wheels from antique farm equipment. Mom found creative ways to use assorted iron pots and kettles for planters. The old junk added a country charm to our yard and garden. Now, as a grown woman, I chuckle when I visit garden shops and see the extravagant price tags on old farm junk.

Beauty by Design

A garden has a beauty all its own—in every season. And as a woman, you are beautiful by design—in every season also. But something in the female spirit loves to add that finishing touch. Every yard and garden nursery offers ornaments, statues, fountains, gnomes, angels, bird baths and more. It can delight and sometimes overwhelm a gardener.

When the hard work of gardening is done, it's refreshing to add a touch of whimsy and beauty. Each garden, like its gardener, has its own personality. The finishing touch for one may be a rustic bird house while for another it may be a marble fountain or statue.

Aren't women just like that? Don't you enjoy adding an adornment to your personal gardens as well? You diet with determination, sweat at the gym and try to get plenty of beauty sleep. Yet with high energy and a soaring spirit, you still enjoy that finishing touch. A favorite of mine is a new pair of earrings. I may feel healthy and fit, but there is nothing quite like new earrings to add sparkle to my outfit *and* life. My Aunt Ruth once told me that she would never wear *old-lady* shoes—even when she became an older woman. Stylish shoes are her crowning touch.

Your Turn...

Complete the following thought-starter:

One of my favorite finishing touches is:

The Outer and Inner Garden United

The décor of your inner wellness garden may appear superficial to some, but many agree that certain finishing touches pay huge health dividends as well as beauty benefits. Three adornments I consider important to the finishing touch of my inner garden are laughter, grace and praise. There certainly are many more ornaments you can select for the health and beauty of your wellness garden, but these, in my opinion, are a great beginning. Let's take a closer look at each of these finishing touches.

There is a fountain of youth: it is your mind, your talents, the creativity you bring to your life and the lives of people you love.
~Sophia Loren, actress

Baskets of Laughter

Volumes of information including statistics and scientific research confirm the health benefits of laughter. We're talking about the roaring, deep belly laughter that brings tears to your eyes and makes your sides ache. Don't you find it interesting that science has to convince some of us to laugh? Recent studies conclude that laughter not only elevates your mood, but improves your immune system, protects your heart, lowers blood pressure, reduces stress and improves brain function.

From a beauty perspective, laughter gives you a glowing countenance and a relaxed appearance. Did you know that smiling uses fewer facial muscles than frowning? Laughter connects you to others, and perhaps that is the greatest value of all.

**You don't stop laughing when you grow old,
you grow old when you stop laughing.**
~George Bernard Shaw

The Grace-filled Woman

Just hearing the word "grace" creates an image of a woman I would love to become. The word is defined as "beauty or charm of form, movement or expression; displaying goodwill or favor, elegance and courtesy." The adornment of grace, gracefulness or graciousness produces an admirable and desirable quality in any woman. This is not a decoration to be "slipped on or off" but one to be cultivated, protected and worn in every season.

The finishing touch of grace may take some work, but the reward of an abundant harvest is guaranteed. Those who are watching you as your inner garden develops will notice the external expressions of grace, and also will feel your inner disposition changing and becoming more beautiful.

When graciousness is strongly rooted in your internal garden, you will shine outwardly with a radiant countenance. A woman adorned (or filled) with grace has the capacity to generously extend gracefulness to others. She brings a spirit of grace into every situation—in every season.

**Cultivate inner beauty, the gentle,
gracious kind that God delights in.**
~1 Peter 3:4

Honor goes to kind and gracious women.
~Proverbs 11:16

Your Turn...

Please complete the following:

The names of some grace-filled women I admire are:

What do I appreciate most about them?

One or two practical ways I can plant grace into my inner garden include:

Praise in the Process

What a joy to hear words of praise for the intentional journey you've taken! Isn't it music to your ears to be commended for your hard work and accomplishments? And rightly so. You worked with determination and commitment to improve your inner garden. Now is the time to reap the well-deserved praise.

I believe that the adornment of praise has two specific benefits that I will mention here. (There are probably many more benefits.) When you are the recipient of praise one benefit is the sense of elated satisfaction in a job well-done or a life well-lived. The second benefit comes when you step beyond yourself to praise others and your Creator God. Praise helps bring everything else together: the planting, the weeding and the harvest. Praise gives a feeling of relief when you've done everything you could then trusted God to provide the harvest.

The woman with praise planted in her heart and on her lips reaps a full harvest in due season. This beautiful finishing touch adds untold blessings to your wellness garden—and perhaps to the gardens of other women as they journey along side you.

We would worry less if we praised more. Thanksgiving is the enemy of discontent and dissatisfaction.
~H.A. Ironside, author

Your Turn...

As you consider the value of praise in your life, please complete the following:

When I receive praise, I feel:

When I give praise, I feel:

Season of Reflection

When I ask women what they want their life story to reveal, most reply that they want their life to be a positive influence for others and that they want to feel valued. Many women express a desire to possess the fruits of purpose and intention, diligence and determination, creativity and conviction.

It takes discipline and courage to blossom into the complete woman you were planted to become—the real you without artificial ingredients—the genuine you that both you and others can love and respect. Becoming the unique woman God designed you to be is worth the risk and the hard work. You *can* become a person who enjoys the privilege and responsibility of taking care of yourself *and* loving those around you.

With time and many back-breaking tasks, the gardener pours her love into both the seeds and soil. She *expects* abundant growth. This same love and expectation planted into your body, mind and spirit produces an abundant harvest of wellness, adorned with laughter, grace and praise. As a result, you blossom into a woman who can live in harmony with her natural rhythms and cycles. You radiate wisdom and a strong sense of confidence. You grow into a woman of wellness through all seasons.

When the world wearies and society ceases to satisfy, there is always the garden.
~Minnie Aumonier, poet

Strolling Down the Garden Path

You've completed the first part of the journey. Congratulate yourself for staying the course. Now that your tools are in order, let's press on. You are on your way to a new beginning!

There is much fruit waiting to be picked and savored. Come with me as we take a look at each season and gather from that season's bountiful, nourishing, and delicious wisdom. This may be your opportunity to experience the seasons in a fresh way.

8

Nature Walk: Learning the Way

The seasons are what a symphony ought to be: four perfect movements in harmony with each other.
—Arthur Rubinstein, 19th century pianist and composer

SEASON IS DEFINED AS "a division of the year as determined by the earth's position with respect to the sun, marked by temperatures, moisture and vegetation." Another definition of the word season is "a period of time or a period of special activity." We see seasons come and go—often without giving them our full attention—sometimes failing to appreciate their provisions or their effect on our health.

A simple understanding of each season's personality helps us savor its gifts and disciplines. One benefit of living wholly in each season is that you may begin your wellness garden whenever you choose. There is no right or wrong time or age to begin cultivating improved health and vitality. Nature has blessed animals in their natural surroundings with an innate wisdom. Their instinct tells them what to eat, when to gather for winter, where to find shelter and when to hibernate. Humans also possess an inner wisdom; we just forget (or neglect) to use it. The more we rely on external conveniences and comforts the less aware we may become of our internal rhythms.

I encourage you to resist how and what the written calendar (and media and marketing experts) urges you to *do* at specific seasons.

For example, we seem to be told when we should make resolutions, lose pounds, take off inches or fight a cold or flu attack. Instead, I suggest you resolve to intentionally and consistently cultivate a wellness lifestyle that honors your body's and Nature's rhythms all year round. Consider the months on the calendar as more than a collection of days. Greet the seasons as different and exciting ways of living! Remember, wellness remains a process, so let's learn as we go and grow—gaining courage, confidence and wisdom along the way—in every personal season.

Life Lessons from a Tree

Perhaps it's because I grew up on the Texas plains (where trees are few and far between) that I feel such an attraction to and affection for every tree I see. I believe trees show us the fullness of the life cycle through all seasons. From the deepest roots to the uppermost branches, the tree offers valuable insight into the relationship between seeds, fruit, falling leaves to bare branches, and our health.

I've chosen illustrations for each of Nature's seasons that show the structure and form of the tree and its similarity to the human body. I believe that the Creator's design of the tree and the human body includes noteworthy similarities. Parallels such as the roots/feet, trunk/body, branches/arms (limbs), sap/blood and fruit/healthy traits fascinate me.

The Chinese Medicine system of health supports the five element theory. This is an impressive approach to nurturing your health and living harmoniously in Nature's seasons. I encourage you to explore this philosophy more deeply. For the purpose of this *Almanac*, I've chosen to focus on those five seasons: Spring, Summer, Late Summer, Fall/Autumn, and Winter. The body's organ groups represented in each of these seasons gives a symbolic reference to the energy and activity associated with those paired organs and their overall effect on your health and healing. In the coming chapters, you will be introduced to these organ groups, their functions and their purpose in a healthy body.

Trees can become damaged and weakened when neglected. Poor soil, dehydration or insect assault can (and often do) greatly reduce *life* in the tree. Your beautiful body desires careful tending and attention as does the tree.

Though a tree grows so high,
the falling leaves return to the root.
~Malay Proverb

Consider the requirements of the trees or plants in your backyard garden. Every attentive gardener knows the importance of a healthy root system for the strength of the tree and production of abundant fruit. Similarly, your body yearns (and needs) to be strong and healthy at the cellular level.

In the thousands of years that human forms have inhabited this planet, their nutrient requirements have not changed. The impressive human body has not evolved through time to become an organism that can be sustained, much less thrive, on artificial ingredients. You must regularly eat fresh vegetables, fruits, roots, seeds, nuts, and grasses for optimal wellness. The first human "in the beginning," had the same anatomical design that you and I share today. Every organ, gland, bone and tissue of our body needs living food with enzymes to spark life into the cells that make up the whole.

When you carefully tend your body's inherent requests, it will carry you through many seasons without being easily uprooted by the winds of change and the occasional storms of life.

Your Turn...

Close your eyes for a moment and envision your "personal healthy."

How does the *healthy you* transfer to an image of yourself as a tree? What kind of tree would you be? A tall, stately oak—a flowing willow? Journal your thoughts here:

Gifts from the Seasons

Every season presents gifts in one form or another. Hopefully, you are wise enough to notice and accept them. Corresponding to each of the seasons, I've prepared and included a seasonal food list of Nature's produce and several simple recipes to help you become acquainted with the natural offerings around you.

Your grandmother was right all along that eating a variety of wholesome foods provides you with the vitamins, minerals, enzymes, amino acids, fiber, essential fatty acids, and healthy sugars and starches you need to sustain and restore your body. Eating in-season foods pleases your senses and provides flavorful nutrition all year long.

In your effort to cultivate healthy habits, consider carefully your food choices and your reasons for those choices. Food issues that concern and perhaps confuse you as a food consumer seem to grow each year. You may believe you are making wise nutritional choices but become overwhelmed with the inclusion of GMO (Genetically Modified Organisms), or the deluge of chemically concocted manufactured "edibles." I call these **F**ake **O**r **O**verly **D**efiled, **P**rocessed **O**r **R**ancid **N**on-foods (F.O.O.D.P.O.R.N.). Sadly, the USDA food pyramid promotes excessive portions of processed grain "edibles" that make up much of the harmful, empty calorie carbohydrates in our modern diet.

When you choose foods "close-to-nature," you will begin to support the normal functioning of all your body's systems. Your immune system becomes stronger to ward off infection. Your digestive system easily and efficiently completes its processes so nutrients get transported to their next destination. The circulatory, respiratory, endocrine systems down to your genetic expression improve when your choices include Nature's seasonal nutritional, healing gifts.

She who loves a garden learns the lessons of the seasons ... and how life itself adheres to nature's plan.
~Mary Engelbreit, Graphic artist and children's book illustrator

Section Two

Planting a Legacy

In Section Two of *The Wise Woman's Almanac* you'll read about each season (Spring, Summer, Late Summer, Fall/Autumn, and Winter) and how each season relates to your own wellness journey. In the first season, you'll encounter Spring. Before you prepare to enter the Spring section, please take a few moments to become familiar with the Spring Tree Illustration.

At the beginning of each season's chapter you'll find a similar tree illustration. I encourage you to review these colorful illustrations and then make notes of any questions you might wish to explore or health goal you want to achieve. Perhaps you'd like to invite a girlfriend or colleague to join you on this adventure. Relax and enjoy your journey.

Spring

Every Seed Counts~Plant with Purpose

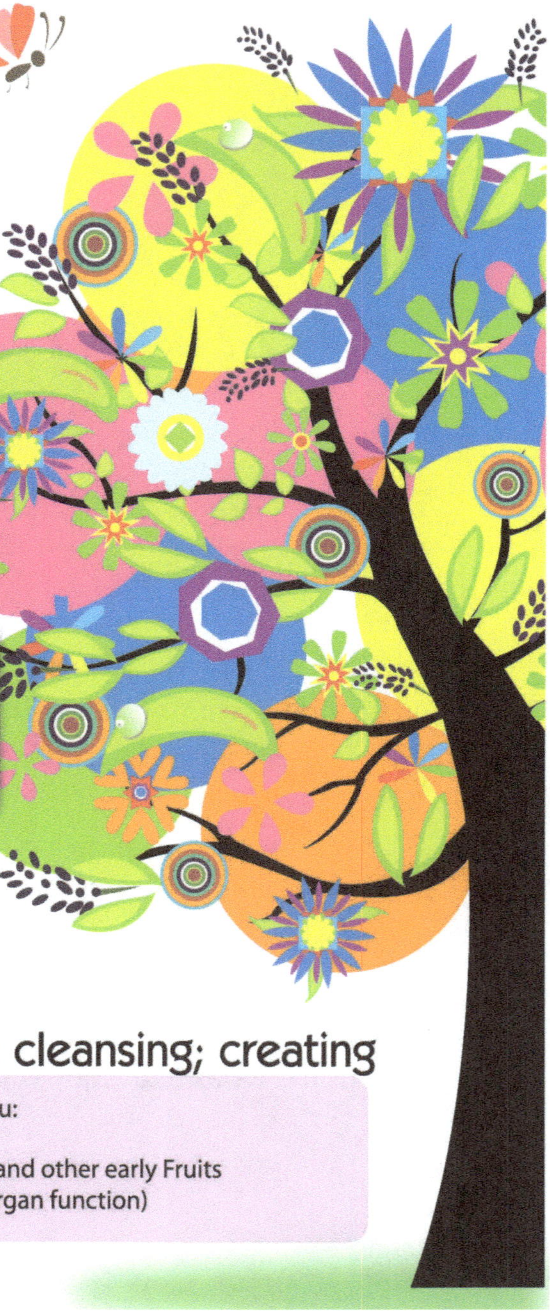

Liver

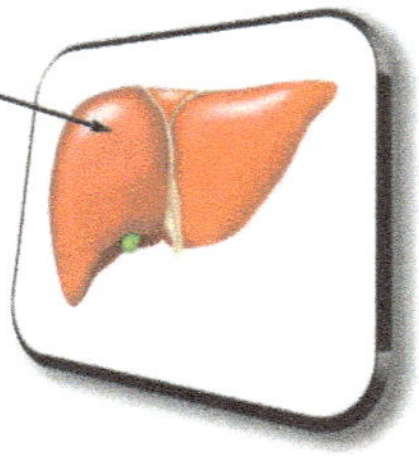

- Largest internal organ assisting 500+ bodily processes

- Affects fat and carbohydrate metabolism

- Plays key role in detoxification

Gall Bladder

- Small pear-shaped organ located behind liver

- Stores bile from liver (necessary for breaking down fats)

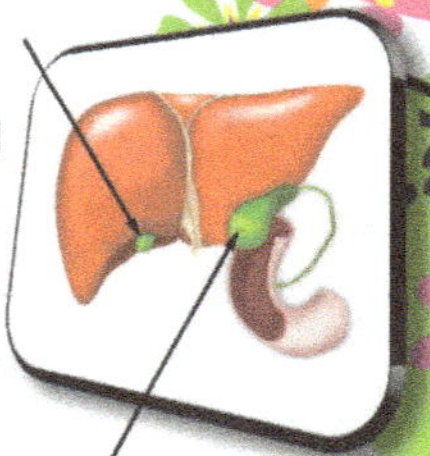

Enlarged Gall Bladder

Season for new beginnings; cleansing; creating

Include these cleansing foods in your Spring menu:

Leafy greens; Sprouts; Bitter herbs, Berries and other early Fruits
Water (hydration is paramount to proper organ function)

9

Spring: Nature's Awakening

In spring time, when the air is calm and pleasant,
it is an injury against nature not to go out, and see her riches,
and partake in her rejoicing with heaven and earth.
—John Milton, 17th century English author

New Life

"Oh, hurry, hurry!" I squeal, as my sister and I run to the chicken house. "I can't wait to see the baby chicks." We breathe in that fresh straw smell as Mom opens the boxes we just received from the hatchery. Little yellow tufts scurry in every direction. Chirping and cheeping, scratching and pecking, the chicks signal the arrival of Spring on the farm.

I fondly remember the many ways Spring announced her coming. Following a long and often harsh Winter, we welcomed every emerging sign of new life! Lilac bushes on the south side of our house served as a fragrant wind break. Robins gathered straw and twigs for their nests. Fruit trees blossomed in sweet smelling pastels—a promise of Summer fruit to come. Tadpoles seemed to appear from nowhere following early rains. Springtime on the farm brought new growth—puppies, kittens, calves, ducks and chicks—always keeping my sister and me happily occupied.

Following Winter's long rest, Nature comes back to life at Springtime. Now is the time to emerge from the indoor comforts of Winter and clean away the wintry residue. It is time for life to sprout, produce and break forth in full bloom. The official beginning of the Spring season begins on March 20 or 21. For the next few months we will experience longer, warmer and brighter days. Wake up—it's Spring!

Spring Means Green

"Get those tumbleweeds raked in a pile, then we'll burn 'em when the wind dies down," Dad instructs. Raking is a Spring ritual on the farm. The Winter winds scatter dried weeds all over the farm and wedge them between barns, fences, chicken houses and sheds. "This pile is ready to burn," I yell back at him. I like the hint of green peeking up from the brown earth after I rake away the Winter debris.

As I look back on these childhood experiences, I recall how Winter's snow becomes merely a memory once Spring presses forth with new life. The dead remains of last year's garden can get raked away and discarded. To me, raking the ground is the out-door equivalent of indoor house cleaning. There's a certain virtue in raking as dormant muscles "spring" to life. (I think as I get older, my muscles crawl to life!) At any rate, this is the season of renewal and I relish it.

> **We need spring. We need it desperately and, usually, we need it before God is willing to give it to us.**
> **~Peter Gzowski, *Spring Tonic***

These outward signs appear quite visible, but something else is happening, as well. It is what is taking place in your internal garden. And sadly, sometimes you neglect this changing inner reality. When you do, you miss the wonder of a vital part of your existence—your *body!* Still while you're preoccupied with tending to the outer duties, your internal ecosystem prepares for another season change.

Spring Has Sprung: There's Cleaning to Be Done!

The Standard American Diet—perhaps more aptly stated: the *standard aging diet*—can bring you added inches, pounds, wrinkles, aches, pains, fatigue, inflammation and premature gray hair! A steady regimen of the processed, refined and artificial food that is so common in today's markets will eventually weaken your internal system and fill your body with waste overload.

However, the human body is incredibly designed to be self-cleaning and to uniquely manage toxicity. Sometimes the body develops chronic complaints, yet at other times it only exhibits slight symptoms or none at all. You can become proactive in helping your amazing body work at an optimum level. Let's explore some intentional ways you can assist your body in cultivating internal cleansing during the Spring season.

The liver and gallbladder are the paired organs needing attention in Spring. These organs take care of your body's internal cleansing and detoxifying processes, so it is appropriate to nurture and nourish them during this time of year.

Rejuvenate Your Inner Garden

The gall bladder, an approximately 3-inch long pear-shaped sac resting in back of the liver on your body's right side serves as a reservoir for bile (a secretion of the liver). It is used in digestion and in the breakdown of fats. The gallbladder is vulnerable to dietary fats and cholesterol, which are major contributors to gallstones.

The liver, the body's largest internal organ, is a cone-shaped, two-lobed organ located in the right upper abdomen. Its hundreds of functions are so vital to life that many refer to it as the body's master laboratory.

A few of the liver's many tasks include storing and distributing nourishment for the entire body, assisting in the formation and breakdown of blood, filtering unusable materials (toxins) from the blood, producing bile to aid in digestion and storing bile in the gallbladder for use in the breakdown of fats, creating more than one thousand enzymes necessary for digestion and assimilation, creating and regulating some of the body's hormones and breaking down proteins into amino acids (useable components for proper digestion and assimilation). The list continues, but this gives you an idea of the liver's value to overall well-being.

Spring Tonic

Spring presents the perfect time to review your habits and patterns, giving you the opportunity to visualize them with new awareness. Your food choices should reflect this season—fresh, whole, cleansing, energizing and life-giving. When you eat foods as Nature intended (not from boxes, wrappers or cans), and add adequate exercise and rest, you are on your way to a well-lived Spring season.

Spring is the time to delight in the life of your garden. Each day brings evidence of newness. New growth, new blossoms, new pods and sprouts, new flowers and fruit and even a few edible weeds, provide the perfect Spring tonic.

I love spring anywhere, but if I could choose
I would always greet it in a garden.
~Ruth Stout, gardener, writer

Simplicity in Springtime

As Nature unfolds her newness around you, the temptation to overdo your Springtime activity may creep in like unwanted weeds. Your revived energy may take you down the path of a worn-out-woman if you aren't attentive. Experiencing an internal cleanse can help you stay balanced during this season. Most health food stores or holistic health providers offer a variety of internal cleansing supplements or programs. Understanding the process before buying allows you to wisely choose the plan best suited for your body and your lifestyle.

Choosing a simple Spring cleanse often brings rewards as great as a lengthy, more involved cleansing process. An internal cleanse can be as simple as a cup of warm water with freshly squeezed lemon juice and one-half of a teaspoon of locally grown honey. This is a great way to begin your day. A lemon offers great therapeutic value following a heavy winter diet of high fat and high protein.

You may decide that a gentle one or two day cleanse will be your next step. You can increase the length of time as your body and mind accept and adapt to this new seasonal ritual. Choose your days with minimal activities planned so your energy will be used efficiently for your cleanse. Plan and prepare to drink fresh fruit and vegetable juices and broths. These may be prepared in a juice machine or purchased from an organic juice vendor. This period without eating solid foods gives the digestive and detoxifying organs time to rest, repair and rebuild.

Another internal cleansing method requires a temporary removal of all—or at least most—non-food items from your diet. The *No White Flour, White Sugar, White Rice or Pasta elimination diet* produces amazing results. These highly refined ingredients are devoid of nutrients and so they create internal deficiencies and contribute to inflammatory conditions. Many of my clients noticed a marked reduction in their body's discomforts when they removed these white items from their diet for a minimum of two weeks. This cleansing plan allows for pure, simple and seasonal foods—just as Nature grew them—prepared simply and healthfully. Raw, steamed, baked or grilled fruits, vegetables and lean protein provide the necessary nutrients without the overload of processed, additive laden and lifeless foods. Once health and vitality were restored, few women cared to return to poor dietary choices and nutrient-deficient foods.

Now that you've become more acquainted with some of Spring's characteristics, let's go to the garden and gather the goodness of this season.

You've got to make a conscious choice every day to shed the old—whatever "the old" means for you.

~Sarah Ban Breathnach, author of *Seasonal Pastimes of the Victorian Home*

10

Nature's Springtime Pantry: Fresh and Clean

Comes the fresh Spring in all her green completed.
—Elizabeth Barrett Browning, 1806-1861, English poet

SPRING FOODS BRING A light, fresh, crisp, fragrant element to the menu. Fruits and berries (now in season) provide vitamins, minerals, water and energy, which enhance the natural internal cleansing process. Greens, a traditional Springtime food choice in most cultures, provide a refreshing, cooling and cleansing effect to the body. Chlorophyll, the green pigment in plants, is considered one of the most powerful healing and cleansing foods known to mankind.

I hope the following list will encourage you to try new foods and bring variety to your table and your body during your next Spring season. Enjoy!

Artichoke (globe)

- A perennial; grows best in cool (not freezing) climates; most abundant in March, April and May; the globe artichoke is different from the Jerusalem artichoke
- Low in calories, high in complex carbohydrates and roughage, an alkaline food
- Contains Vitamins A and C, calcium, iron and inulin (a starch that helps improve blood sugar imbalances in diabetics), reduces

cholesterol, supports liver/gall bladder, stimulates bile, enhances digestion and detoxifies

Asparagus

- A perennial; member of the lily family; peak season is April, May, June
- Green variety is higher in nutrients due to chlorophyll content
- Low in calories and carbohydrates, high in protein, and is alkaline
- Acts as a stimulant to the kidneys; acts as a blood purifier when taken in moderation

Avocado

- Actually a fruit with over 400 varieties; consumed more often as a vegetable than a fruit; complements both fruit and vegetable dishes
- High in quality protein and unsaturated fatty acids (oleic and linoleic) that are easily digested and assimilated for an exceptional energy food; is an alkaline food

Beets

- Roots and leaves (greens) are both edible
- Beneficial for every organ in the body—especially the liver, gallbladder, digestive and lymphatic systems and the bowels
- Provide high content organic mineral salts that aid in tissue repair, detoxify the blood and circulate nutrients to every cell in the body
- Good source of betain (brain food), folate (anti-depression B-vitamin), amino acids (glutamine and asparagine)
- High in iron, antioxidants, flavonoids, beta carotene, ascorbic acid, calcium, potassium, Vitamins A and C

- Greens are exceptionally high in chlorophyll, flavonoids and carotenes
- Recommended in anti-cancer and heart health diets

Carrot

- Member of celery, parsnip, caraway, fennel, parsley, dill and chervil family
- Available year round; considered the "king of vegetables"
- Rich source of pro-vitamin A, protein, calcium, iron, vitamins B and C and is alkaline

Celery

- Available year round with its peak season from November through May
- High in silicon (aids in renewal of bone, joints, arteries and connective tissue), potassium, Vitamin C and fiber
- Contains substances that relax smooth muscle lining of blood vessels (improving hypertension), high in water content and is alkaline

Cruciferous Group

- Cool season crops with peak season from late Fall to early Spring
- Includes broccoli, Brussels sprouts, cabbage, cauliflower, collard greens, cress, horseradish, kale, kohlrabi, mustard, radish, rutabaga and turnip with similar healing properties in all varieties
- Rich in minerals, cancer fighting phytochemicals; sulfur content improves circulation; nutrients benefit respiratory, digestive, lymphatic, urinary, skeletal and elimination systems of the body

Grapefruit

- A subtropical fruit with an alkaline action in the body; peak season is January through May.
- Its sweet and sour taste improves poor digestion, reduces intestinal gas, promotes healthy bowel action and removes mucus from the lungs.
- Grapefruit Seed Extract is well known for its effective antibiotic properties in reducing various bacteria and virus.
- Rich in vitamins C, B1 and B2, potassium and flavonoids; low in calories; has less sugar than an orange; is less acidic than a lemon.

Greens

- Often referred to as a common weed, greens add many necessary nutrients to the diet.
- Darker greens are higher in calcium, magnesium and chlorophyll (helps regulate calcium in body). High chlorophyll content helps cleanse blood, acts as tonic for brain and immune system and promotes healthy intestinal flora.
- Common early Spring greens include chard, chickweed, chicory, cilantro, dandelion, and parsley.

Lettuce

- Cool weather crop; common varieties include butterhead, leaf lettuce, stem lettuce, romaine and spinach.
- Contains Vitamins A, C, E, B-complex, calcium and iron (darker greens contain higher iron).

Mint

- Peppermint and Spearmint are best known varieties.
- Used for indigestion, heartburn, fever, headache, motion sickness and antispasmodic.

- Other members of the mint family include basil, lemon balm, marjoram, sage, savory, oregano, rosemary and thyme.

Onion

- Member of the lily family which also includes chives, garlic, leek, scallion, and shallot.
- Pungency from the amino acid, allicin, helps promote flow of digestive and immune fluids, removing mucus and purifying the blood.

Orange

- Available year round, with the U.S. peak season from January through May.
- High in flavonoids (plant pigment providing excellent protection from free-radical damage).
- Healing properties include immune system support, strengthening the connective tissue, lowering cholesterol, improving sluggish digestive tract and improving acidic conditions in the body.

Peas

- A frost hardy, cool season crop, with the peak season from March to July.
- Alkaline, with a complete source of incomplete protein (more easily digestible than beans).
- Excellent source of Vitamins A, B1 and C. The pods are high in chlorophyll, iron and insoluble fiber.
- Varieties include English peas, Snap peas, and Snow peas (sugar peas).
- The Southern pea (cowpea) is a warm weather crop grown similarly to beans.

Pineapple

- Available year round, most abundant from April to July.
- Excellent source of bromelain (enzyme that increases digestive ability and has anti-inflammatory properties).
- Great for quenching thirst and relieving sunstroke.
- Ripe pineapple is juicy and sweet and not acidic.
- Acts as diuretic and digestive aid (not to be consumed if peptic ulcer or skin discharge is present).

Rhubarb

- Member of the sorrel family (bitter greens), grown in cooler regions.
- Beneficial in lowering cholesterol, dissolving intestinal mucus, reducing liver toxicity (especially over consumption of meat) and acting as a mild laxative.
- Good source of fiber and Vitamin C.
- Because of extreme bitter flavor, it mixes well with apples, plums or strawberries.

Herbs: Medicine from the Garden

Spring's warming temperatures begin to thaw the hardened ground of Winter producing splashes of green around your yard or garden. Unfortunately, in our Western culture, too many consumers spend much time and money trying to rid their outdoor space of these "weeds." Did you know that those obnoxious weeds in your garden may be giving you a message about the condition (imbalances) of the soil in your yard?

I learned from Steven Horn, an herbalist and instructor at the School of Modern Herbal Medicine, that different weeds thrive in different soil conditions. Certain weeds thrive in compact soil because their growth loosens the soil. Some weeds actually balance soil deficiencies while other weeds grow well in toxic soils because they tend to detoxify the soil.

Horn suggests learning the nature of the weeds, then treating or balancing the soil and the weeds usually will bid your yard or garden good-bye.

A weed is a plant whose virtues have not yet been discovered.
~Ralph Waldo Emerson

I love the similarities between Nature's earth and my body. Along the path of my personal wellness journey I've discovered that healing principles are also similar.

The use of plants as medicine dates back to the beginning of time. Those ancient native cultures I mentioned in previous chapters found many healing and medicinal uses for seasonal weeds, more lovingly known as herbs. Many of our modern medicines have their roots, so to speak, in plants.

Whether you choose to use herbs as a healing tool for your wellness journey or as a culinary herb to bring flavorful life to your recipes, I invite you to get acquainted with this simple, beginner's list of Spring-into-Summer Herbs. Enjoy!

Alfalfa

- Regarded as the "Father of all foods" due to its high content of easily digested vitamins, minerals, (iron, calcium, magnesium, phosphorous, sulfur, chlorine, sodium, potassium, silicon), trace minerals and protein (contains eight of the essential amino acids)
- Commonly used for conditions pertaining to arthritis, digestive distress, elevated cholesterol levels, halitosis and body odor (chlorophyll is a natural deodorizer)

- Enjoyed best as sprouts (from seeds) or as a tea (from the dried plant).

Aloe

- Traditionally used externally for the treatment of skin burns (sun, wind, fire, chemical), cuts, abrasions and poisonous plant irritations.
- The inner leaf gel is a beneficial skin moisturizer and is an ingredient in many skin care products.
- Aloe vera juice, taken internally effectively soothes digestive disorders and improves inflamed gut lining tissue due to aloe's ability to promote cellular growth and repair.

Basil

- From the Greek word, King, this aromatic herb relieves stomach discomforts (cramping or nausea) and relieves intestinal gas.
- As a culinary herb, basil lends a heady, warm flavor to Italian or Mediterranean style dishes; finely chopped, it adds flavor and color to appetizers, dips, sauces, egg and cheese dishes, and squash or tomato dishes.

Capsicum/Cayenne

- Nutritional and medicinal, this herb improves the metabolism and stimulates circulation.
- Contains more Vitamin C than oranges, iron, calcium phosphorous, and the B-Vitamins.
- Soothes indigestion; reduces inflammation; relieves congestion and improves immunity.
- This spicy pepper adds zest to any dish, so use sparingly; you'll not want to get this near your eyes.

Chives

- Member of the lily family; high in Vitamin C and iron.
- Improves anemia and digestion.
- Add this mild, onion flavored herb, freshly chopped, to potatoes, soups, sauces, seafood; add to softened butter for delightful herb butter spread.

Cilantro

- Commonly used as a detoxifying herb; effective in cleansing metal toxicity from the body's tissues; it has been called, "the poor man's chelation" remedy.
- Rich source of healing phytonutrients and antioxidants, Vitamins A, C, K and some B-Vitamins; provides calcium, potassium, iron, manganese and sodium.
- Reduces anxiety; promotes efficient bowel activity; excellent blood builder, preventing anemia; acts as a natural diuretic helping to reduce or prevent kidney stones; anti-inflammatory.
- The fantastic flavor pairs well with many foods but especially Mexican dishes; add freshly chopped cilantro to soups, salads, sauces and salsas.

Dandelion

- Perennial herb used mostly as greens; considered a weed by many gardeners.
- Provides wealth of vitamins, minerals, protein, choline, pectins and carotenoids.
- Best known for its liver cleansing and toning properties .
- All parts of the plant are edible (roots, leaves, blossoms), and may be taken steeped as a tea, snipped into green salads or smoothies or added to jellies, jams or wine (blossoms).

Dill

- With a long history of health benefits, dill protects against free radical damage; provides plentiful sources of Vitamins A and C, and the minerals calcium, magnesium, iron, copper, potassium and manganese.
- Common uses include relief for digestive discomforts; stimulates milk production in nursing mothers; soothes nervous conditions.
- A popular herb in European and Mediterranean dishes; freshly snipped dill pairs well with cheese, salads, soups and is used in pickling recipes.

Garlic

- A perennial herb (in the onion and chive family), known as "Nature's antibiotic" and is used for fighting infection (bacterial, viral, fungal, staphylococcus and E. coli).
- Supports heart health, modulates cholesterol levels and helps emulsify plaque on arterial walls.
- Restores and rejuvenates cellular function; promotes endurance and energy.
- The robust flavor of fresh garlic enhances many types of foods, especially Italian and Mediterranean dishes.

Horseradish

- A powerhouse of nutrients providing cancer protection and healing properties for respiratory disorders or congestion, fevers, sinusitis and coughs.
- This pungent plant is related to mustard, cabbage and wasabi; used in appetizer dips, cocktail sauces, relishes, salad dressings and a condiment on meats.

Oregano

- Greek for "mountain joy," this aromatic herb provides antioxidant, antibacterial and anti-inflammatory properties that improve respiratory, gastrointestinal and urinary disorders.
- High in iron, Vitamin E and K, calcium, manganese and omega fatty acids this herb promotes healthy bone growth and density and the production of blood clotting proteins.
- Culinary uses include Mexican and Mediterranean cuisines, soup, stew, stuffing seasoning, and pasta sauces.

Parsley

- High in Vitamins A, C, and some B's and the minerals calcium, copper, iron, manganese and potassium, parsley stimulates the immune system and increases the body's resistance to disease.
- The diuretic properties make this a beneficial kidney and bladder herb; helps calm digestion after eating and is soothing for respiratory irritation.
- The flat-leaf or curly variety may be used in any green drink or in stuffings, egg dishes or toppings on grilled meat.

Peppermint – Spearmint

- A rich source of nutrients including Vitamin C, manganese, copper offering antioxidant and anti-inflammatory properties.
- Widely used to soothe symptoms of indigestion including irritable bowel or colitis; contains plant compounds that improve respiratory conditions (asthma, bronchitis), and sinus related allergies.
- Commonly steeped as a tea (hot or cold); flavoring for candy; used in Asian and Middle Eastern cooking.

Rosemary

- Most commonly used for its memory improving properties and relief of headaches and nervous tension; improves immune function and circulatory system.
- A good source of iron, calcium and Vitamin B6.
- The bold and piney flavor enhances breads, meat and fish, soups, sauces, rice, and vegetable dishes.

Sage (garden)

- Rich source of several B-vitamins, Vitamin A and beta-carotene, Vitamin C and the minerals potassium, zinc, calcium, iron, manganese, copper and magnesium.
- The fresh leaves add a flavorful addition to stuffings, roasted pork or lamb; also used to flavor vegetable dishes especially with beans.

Thyme

- Rich in Vitamins A, C, iron, copper, manganese, and dietary fiber.
- Powerful antioxidant properties improve respiratory function, ease congestion in chest and head; has a soothing sedative action on nervous conditions; reduces fevers.
- The slightly minty flavor is an excellent seasoning in poultry or seafood dishes, creamy soups, chowders and sauces, stews and stuffings; often paired with tomatoes.

Connie's Comments: Most of these simple garden herbs grow well in pots, planters or small containers making it easy for you to "grow-your-own." If you do purchase fresh herbs, you'll want to select locally grown, when possible, chemical free and organic herbs. If you desire to use Nature's foods for therapeutic reasons, please consult a professional in herbal medicine or check with your professional health provider for appropriate and effective dosages. There may be plant (herb) interactions or contraindications with medications you may be currently taking, so please research first! In rare cases, plant allergies may be a consideration. If you have plant allergies, please review the plant family and botanical properties before using an herb for the first time.
I encourage and support wellness with wisdom!

11

Nature's Springtime Recipes: Refreshing and Energizing

The greatest gift of the garden is the restoration of the five senses.
—Hanna Rion (1875-1924) landscape illustrator

Cleansing Green Juice Cocktail

An easy to prepare juice to use anytime you feel like doing a short cleanse or fast, this juice provides vitamins. minerals and fiber, using cleansing vegetables and herbs. Green drinks often taste bitter, but this promotes digestive activity and the cleansing process. Wash produce thoroughly. *(The recipe for a homemade fresh produce wash follows this juice recipe.)*

- 1 stalk celery, cut in 1-inch pieces
- 2-3 sprigs curly parsley
- 2-3 dandelion leaves
- 3-4 beet top greens
- 1 medium apple, cored and cut in wedges
- 1/2 medium lemon, cut in 1-inch pieces

Place all ingredients in juicing machine container.
Add 2 cups water.
Blend until all ingredients are well blended. Add more water to reach desired consistency.
Season with sea salt and freshly ground pepper if desired.
Drink about 3/4 - 1 cup. Remaining green juice may be stored in refrigerator for 1-2 days.

Connie's Comments: If dandelion leaves or beet tops are not available, you may substitute 2-3 leaves romaine lettuce. If you prefer a sweeter taste, add 1/4 cup freshly sliced (not canned) pineapple.

Fresh Produce Wash

Thorough washing of fresh fruits and vegetables rids the surface of untold contaminants (pesticides, waxes, human handling) and insures a safer and tastier food as well as a prolonged storage. The Environmental Working Group reports that a simple white vinegar and water wash kills 98 percent of surface bacteria as well as removes residue from wax coatings and pesticides.

Sink Soak Recipe

- Fill your kitchen sink or a large bowl with purified room temperature water (tap water contains contaminants).
- Add white vinegar in a 1-3 ratio (1-part white vinegar to 3-parts water).
- Add 1-Tbsp. salt and swish water with hands to dissolve the salt.
- Place your fresh (room temperature) produce in the water, washing the more delicate produce first (berries, leafy greens); soak produce for about 10 minutes; gently remove to a colander or strainer and rinse; place on paper towels on a clean counter or drip tray to air dry before storing.
- Repeat the process with heartier produce (celery, kale, potatoes, etc.).

Spray Wash Recipe

- Slice one lemon in half and squeeze 1-Tbsp. of its juice into a measuring cup.
- Add 2-Tbsp. baking soda to the lemon juice.
- Add 1-cup purified water to the lemon juice-baking soda mixture.

- Whisk briskly so that baking soda completely dissolves into the lemon juice and water.
- Pour this mixture into a clean spray bottle.
- Place your fresh produce in a colander/strainer in the kitchen sink.
- Spray produce with lemon wash to completely coat outer surface; let fresh produce "sit" in wash for about 10 minutes.
- Rinse thoroughly with clean water; place clean produce on paper towels or drip tray to air dry before storing.

Roasted Asparagus

Serves 8
Prep Time: 30 minutes

Roasting concentrates the flavor of asparagus and gives the spears a firm, crunchy texture

3 pounds asparagus, trimmed
3 Tbsp. olive oil

- Preheat oven to 400°F; Toss asparagus with oil on baking sheet (I line the baking sheet with parchment paper) and season with salt and pepper.
- Roast 10 minutes or until asparagus are tender; turn spears to roast other side for about 2-4 more minutes. Turn oven off.
- Remove baking tray from oven; arrange asparagus on serving platter.

Connie's Comments: I like to sprinkle freshly grated Parmesan cheese on top of the asparagus in the last 2-4 minutes of roasting for a bit of crunch. Sea salt and freshly ground pepper may be used for additional seasoning, if desired. Sliced almonds may also be added for a crunchy topping as an alternative to the Parmesan cheese.

Spring Pea and Bean Salad

Serves 4

1 cup fresh or frozen edamame, shelled
1 cup fresh or frozen green peas
1 cup fresh or frozen lima beans
Zest and juice of 1 small lemon (about 1 teaspoon zest and 2-1/2 teaspoons juice)
3 Tbsp. white wine vinegar
2 green onions, minced
2 Tbsp. chopped fresh mint
1 Tbsp. chopped fresh chives
¼ cup extra virgin olive oil
Sea salt and freshly ground pepper to taste
1 ounce pecorino cheese, shaved

- In medium saucepan, cook edamame in steamer basket about 2 minutes or until crisp-tender. Remove with a wire-mesh strainer, and plunge beans into ice water to stop the cooking process; drain and set aside. Return water to a boil; add peas, and cook about 4 minutes, repeating draining process. Repeat with lima beans, cooking about 5 minutes.
- Combine lemon zest and juice, wine vinegar, onions, mint, chives in a small bowl. Gently whisk in oil until well blended. Season with salt and pepper.
- Place peas and beans in a medium bowl and toss with vinaigrette. Top with pecorino, and garnish with fresh mint, if desired.

Connie's Comment: Whenever I steam or boil vegetables, I follow my grandmother's health secret and save the boiling water to drink once it is cooled. It's full of nutrients!

Garden Herb Salad with Roasted Shallot Vinaigrette

Serves 6

The slightly sweet flavor of the roasted shallot in the vinaigrette dressing balances the bitterness of the mixed spring herbs.

1 medium shallot, peeled
2 Tbsp. red wine vinegar
1 Tbsp. extra virgin olive oil
1 tsp. sugar
1 tsp. Dijon mustard
¼ tsp. salt
¼ tsp. black pepper
1 4-ounce package Spring herb salad mix

- Preheat oven to 375°F.
- Wrap shallot in parchment paper and seal well; Bake for 35 minutes; cool for 10 minutes; Peel and mince.
- Combine shallot, vinegar, oil, sugar, mustard, salt and pepper in large bowl; stir well with a whisk.
- Place salad mix in large serving bowl; Drizzle with vinaigrette; toss well to coat.

Walnut Pear Salad

Serves 4

This nutty salad is absolutely beautiful with mixed greens. Pears and apricot nectar add a fruity sweetness.

1/3 cup apricot nectar
2 Tbsp. olive oil
2 Tbsp. red wine vinegar
1 tsp. chopped fresh mint or l/4 teaspoon dried mint flakes
1/8 tsp. salt
1/8 tsp. ground mustard

3 medium pears, peeled, halved and sliced
12 cups mixed salad greens
¾ cup chopped walnuts, toasted

- In a jar with a tight fitting lid, combine the nectar, olive oil, red wine vinegar, mint, salt and ground mustard; shake well.
- Combine the pears and dressing in a large serving bowl. Cover and refrigerate until chilled.
- Just before serving, add greens to pear mixture; toss to coat.
- Sprinkle with walnuts.

Nourishing Broth

Fill a stock pot with the following washed and chopped vegetables.

2 white potatoes with peeling
4 carrots (tops removed)
4 stalks celery
2 green onions
3-4 cloves garlic
2 small red beets, stems and tops included
Small head broccoli
Leafy greens: (choose 2) Swiss chard, kale, collards, parsley
Bragg Liquid Aminos (for amino acid supplementation)

- Cover vegetables with water, cover pot with lid and bring to a low boil until vegetables are tender.
- Let cool; strain the vegetables OUT of the water and discard (the nutrients have been cooked out of them).
- Bragg Liquid Aminos may be added sparingly for extra flavor. Season the broth to your liking with cayenne or basil, oregano, paprika or cumin.
- The broth may be refrigerated for 2-3 days and used during your spring cleanse/fast.

12

Reflections on the Season: Spring Forward

Despite the forecast, live like it's spring!
—Lilly Pulitzer, author

Your Turn ...

To help you understand how you are in Spring *and how* Spring is in you, *I invite you to complete these following thought-starters:*

My favorite childhood memories of Spring are:

My favorite Spring activity is:

My favorite Spring foods/recipes are:

In Springtime I feel:

My thoughts on Spring are:

Before you read about how Summer affects your physical, emotional and spiritual life, I invite you to spend a few moments looking at the Summer Tree Illustration. Familiarize yourself with the organ group and list of Summer foods that can enhance your health.

Summer

Healthy Roots Produce Healthy Fruit

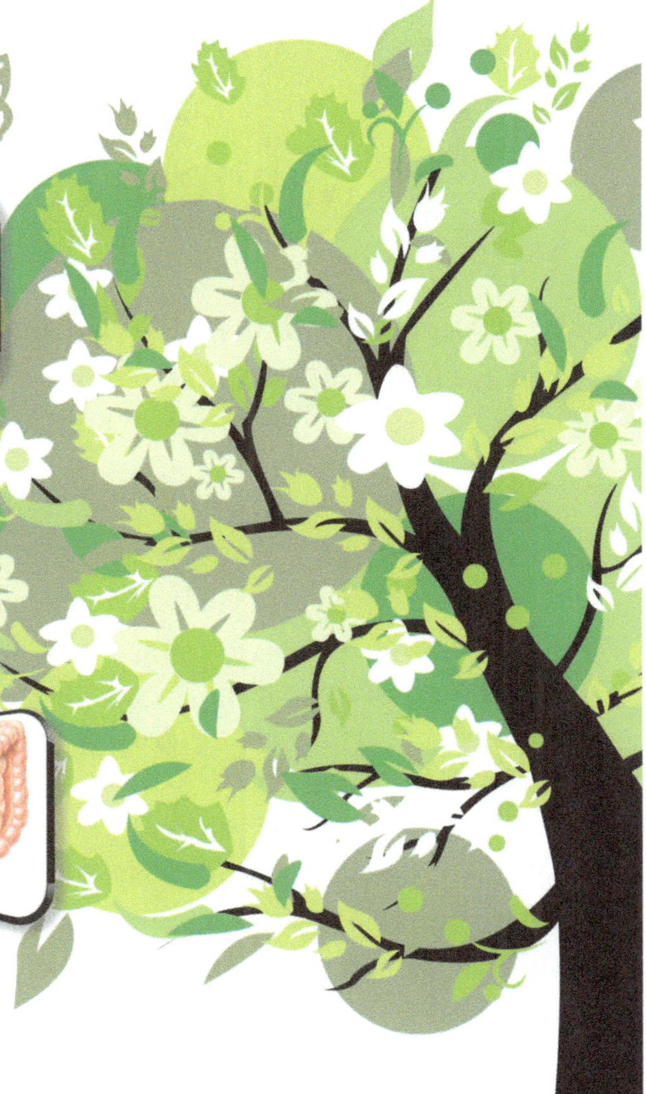

Heart

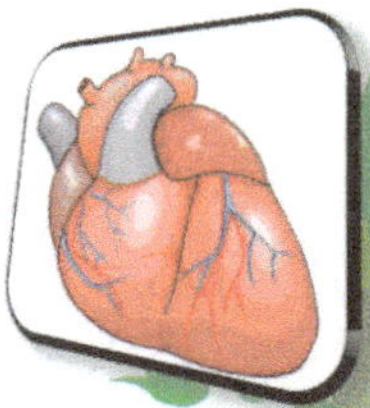

- Circulates blood to transport oxygen to the cells and remove cellular wastes

- Four-chambered pump circulating 3,000-gallons of blood per day

Small Intestine

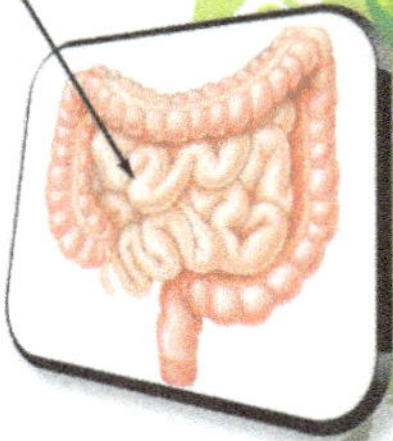

- Long, narrow tubing from stomach to large intestine that collects, digests and assimilates food

- Plays key role in fat and carbohydrate digestion

- Separates nutrients from wastes, then transports nutrients to the blood

Season of Increased Activity and Energy

Include these cooling foods in your Summer menu:

Cucumber, Watermelon, Fresh fruits, Summer squash, and other vine-ripened fresh produce
Water (hydration cools the body's internal temperature and aids digestion)

13

Summer: Nature in Full Bloom

Summer is not so much a season as a melody, that tune of contentment we hum as the days begin to beautifully blur.
—Sarah Ban Breathnach, author

"I'M NEXT! I'M NEXT," CALLS my sister. Youthful laughter fills the sultry afternoon as we run through the sprinkler. The neighbor kids join us in the cool, wet fun as we try to beat the Texas heat. "Hey, Lucky wants to play too," I say, watching our soggy little spaniel jump through the sprays of water. Summertime on the farm is a busy time, and I welcome the chance to *play*.

Summer in the Texas Panhandle blows in hot and dry. Even with the unpleasant climate, many of my favorite memories come from that time. Sunday afternoons usually meant homemade ice cream. I felt grown up when Dad let me turn the crank on the ice cream maker. Running through the wide open spaces of our farm and catching June bugs between eating bites of ice cream brought the perfect end to a hot summer's day.

June 21st marks the arrival of Summer. Most school schedules have taken a Summer break and swimming pools await the throngs of sun worshippers. As Oscar Hammerstein II wrote in 1945, "June is bustin' out all over."

Summer's rhythms appear all around as the earlier sunrises and later sunsets bring indescribable colors for a visual delight. Fragrant ripened fruit and vegetables and freshly mowed grass offer aromatic pleasures. My childhood Summers also brought wheat harvest, one of my favorite seasonal activities. Those flat Texas plains turned golden with ripening wheat in the hot sun and breezes. That often irritating sensation of hot wind blowing against the skin and messing the hair reminds us that Summer has arrived.

Deep Roots

Looking back on my farming beginnings, I observe a connection between the harshness and the strength of the Summer months. The trees—what few there are on the Texas plains—hold strong in the Summer's windy heat. Garden crops and yard shrubbery grow stout to withstand the daily fifteen to twenty miles per hour "breezes." It amused my husband on his first visit to my family's farm to see all the trees leaning north.

Summer also brings tornado season, when Nature fiercely demonstrates her power. Developing strong roots, in spite of the often daily weather adversity, proved valuable to those Texas trees. Likewise, it's important for us to cultivate a strong and healthy internal root system in order to withstand the difficulties life sometimes throws at us. Summertime, with its climate extremes, offers the perfect growing season to tend to our inner roots. Once again, our beautiful body responds to seasonal change. Learning to care for our body's Summer needs directly affects how well it will function in the Fall/Autumn and Winter.

To be rooted is perhaps the most important and least recognized need of the human soul.
~Simone Weil, French philosopher

Health in Summer's Heat

The organs of the body that are associated with Summer include the heart and small intestine. I want to share with you how these organs work together for optimal wellness during the hot Summer season.

The small intestine is part of the digestive system. About twenty-two feet in length, it nestles between the stomach and large intestine (colon). The primary functions of the small intestine are to receive, digest and absorb nutrients. Very simply, it sorts the necessary from the *un*-necessary. Nutrients pass directly to the blood supply and wastes move to the large intestine for elimination. I wish my house could be so self-cleaning!

If (for any number of reasons such as illness, injury, stress, or poor diet) the small intestine becomes unable to fulfill its natural functions effectively, incomplete digestion may result. This often produces an overly acidic condition in the body. Once weakened, the entire digestive system can become vulnerable to digestive disorders and possibly more serious conditions. The Standard American Diet of highly processed and refined foods greatly contributes to excessive acid and inflammation in the small intestine. From the vast number of digestive aid advertisements, it appears that many Americans suffer from chronic digestive disorders.

Your Body's Second Brain

New and exciting studies on the small intestine identify the gut (large and small intestines) as the body's second brain. The condition of the gut profoundly influences your overall health. Revolutionary new research suggests that the gastrointestinal system mirrors the brain in producing major neurotransmitters, including serotonin, as well as several hormones. Serotonin produces a calming effect on the digestive tract and initiates healthy gut function. This new knowledge in gut health and overall well-being, especially for conditions like anxiety and depression, presents exciting possibilities in better understanding the connection between food and mood.

David Perlmutter, MD, a Board-Certified Neurologist and Fellow of the American College of Nutrition, explains that your brain's health is dictated by what goes on in your gut. Did you ever think that the gurgling in your gut might affect your perceptions of life? Or be at the root of your migraine headache? Or even restrict your energy or libido?

Dr. Perlmutter also recommends including a diet rich in probiotic and prebiotic foods. Probiotic foods include:

- Fermented/pickled fruits and vegetables (sauerkraut, pickles, etc.)
- Yogurt/kefir with active bacteria (healthy) cultures
- Kimchi and cultured condiments

Recommended prebiotic foods include:

- Raw garlic, onion (also cooked), leek
- Raw asparagus
- Raw dandelion greens, chicory root
- Raw banana

Taking care of your small intestine (gut) promotes well-rooted physical and emotional health for many seasons.

Digestion, of all the bodily functions, is the one which exercises the greatest influence on the mental state of an individual.
~Jean-Anthelme Brillat-Savarin, 1755-1826, Food Critic and Author

Heart of the Matter

The heart is the second organ considered in Summer. This fist-sized, hollow, muscular double-pump is the center of the circulatory system. Just as the sap of a tree circulates water and nutrients to the upper branches, the heart circulates oxygen and nutrients to all parts of your body.

The heart, located in the center of the chest and behind the sternum (chest bone), tilts slightly to the left. It beats between 60 to 80 times per minute in most people or about one hundred thousand times per day. Your entire blood supply passes through your heart every sixty seconds. The right and left sides of the heart pump blood in two different directions, moving oxygen and nutrients to the cells and wastes out of the cells. While that process is in motion, the heart also keeps the body's temperature in balance.

Phrases such as broken-hearted, hard-hearted, tender-hearted, cold-hearted, faint-hearted, half-hearted and heart-felt are not medical terms, yet they express the emotional essence of a person's heart, the most essential internal organ. Psychoneuroimmunology, the science that demonstrates how emotional conditions affect heart rate, function, artery health and immune response, helps us understand the body-mind-spirit connection.

Sadly, cardiovascular disease steps up as the number one killer of American women. It usually strikes via a heart attack or stroke and claims nearly 500,000 women each year. Now is the time to tend the garden of your heart. And you would be wise to heed the lessons of Summer in taking care of your heart. Summer's naturally cooling foods support healthy heart function for an active life through many seasons.

Everyone is the age of their heart.
~Guatemalan Proverb

Play It Cool

Data collected by the Environmental Protection Agency suggests that hot weather extremes have a greater effect on mortality than cold weather. Humidity is another important factor in mortality since it contributes to the body's ability to cool itself through evaporation of perspiration.

Heat affects mood changes, often contributing to higher incidences of aggression. Warmer temperatures increase the body's metabolism, which provides energy for Summer activities and for shedding unwanted winter weight. Many factors influence the health of the human body. A simple understanding of how your body works under normal conditions helps prepare you for seasonal changes. In order to allow your body to digest completely and cool down during the sweltering days of Summer, plan to take adequate rest periods, consume lighter meals and drink sufficient amounts of water.

As I mentioned in Chapter 6, under Water Wisdom, the controversy continues among the experts on the recommended daily intake of water. It is vital to your health to observe your body's signals and drink enough water per day to provide for the moderately active body's hydration needs.

The LORD watches over you—the LORD is your shade at your right hand; the sun will not harm you by day, nor the moon by night.

~Psalm 121:5-6

14

Nature's Summer Pantry: Cool Foods for Hot Days

There is a remedy for every illness to be found in nature.
—Hippocrates, the Father of Medicine

YOU'LL RARELY EXPERIENCE A boring meal when you use fresh, sun-ripened Summer produce for your recipes. Nature encourages a healthy lifestyle in Summer with an abundance of ripe and ready crops. Farmers' markets thrive in Summer and many communities are fortunate to have local growers sell their produce during this beautiful growing season. I suggest you visit your local farmers' market often and purchase some of the following seasonal fruits and vegetables. Then you'll be able to savor the flavor and variety that this Summer list offers.

Apple

- Available year round in numerous varieties.
- Alkaline, containing pectin (acts as soft bulking agent in intestine).
- Contains 50 percent more Vitamin A than oranges; abundant in Vitamin C and Vitamin B (maintains nerve health) and has a moderate supply of iron.

Apricot

- A summer fruit; only 20 percent of harvest is sold as fresh fruit—mostly sold as dried, canned or frozen.

- Alkaline; excellent source of Vitamin A, potassium, magnesium, iron and carotenes; has a laxative effect.

Asparagus

- Perennial herb, member of the Lily of the Valley family.
- In-season from February through July, peaking in April, May, June.
- Green variety is higher in nutrients, due to chlorophyll content.
- Alkaline; acts as stimulant to the kidneys; acts as blood builder when taken in moderation.

Avocado

- A fruit with more than 400 varieties.
- Used more often as a vegetable; blends well with fruits or vegetables.
- At its peak, it contains high content of quality protein and unsaturated fatty acids (oleic and linoleic acids); is an exceptional energy food.
- Helps maintain normal cholesterol levels; good source of potassium (heart health).
- Alkaline; source of 13 essential minerals including, iron, copper and magnesium.

Beans – Green

- In season from Summer through early Fall/Autumn; often called string beans.
- High in Vitamins A, C and K; excellent source of calcium, magnesium, iron, phosphorous, potassium, copper, thiamin, niacin, riboflavin, folate, fiber and protein.
- Nutrients protect the heart and colon, reduce inflammation and provide energy.

Beets

- Available year round, with peak season May through October.
- High fiber content favorably affects bowel function, digestive and lymphatic systems, which may contribute to anti-cancer benefits.
- Beet greens contain higher nutrients than the root, containing calcium, iron, Vitamins A and C.

Berries

- Rich in vital nutrients, low in calories (great for that sweet tooth).
- Excellent source of potassium, water soluble fibers, flavonoids (plant pigments providing remarkable protection against free-radical damage).
- Common berries include: blackberry, blueberry, raspberry, strawberry.

Broccoli

- One of the most nutrient dense foods; exceptionally high in Vitamin C.
- One cup serving offers same amount of protein as one cup of rice or corn, but without the calories.
- Contains compounds called indoles, which increase the excretion of estrogen (the type linked with breast cancer).

Carrots

- Rich source of pro-vitamin A carotenes, beneficial to eye health.
- Carrot tops are rich in potassium, but very bitter in taste (finely chop and add to salads or tie in bundle and use for broth flavoring).
- Carrots add roughage as well as nutrients to the diet.

Cherry

- Peak season is June and July.
- Rich source of flavonoids; effective in lowering uric acid levels and preventing gout; reduces inflammatory conditions.
- High in iron; exceptional blood builder and liver and gall bladder cleanser.
- Alkaline; excellent laxative.

Corn

- Actually, corn is a grain.
- Provides complex carbohydrates, essential fatty acids, Vitamin E.
- Peak season is July through September; fresh corn on the cob is high in enzymes and vitamins.
- High in magnesium; regulates bowel activity.

Cucumber

- Alkaline, non-starchy and exceptionally cooling to the body's circulatory system.
- Outer skin is high in silica (mineral that strengthens connective tissue).
- Cucumber juice relieves pain of burns, especially sunburn.

Eggplant

- At their peak from August through October; member of the nightshade family.
- Excellent source of Vitamins B1 and B6, potassium, manganese, copper and fiber.
- Low in calories, they help lower blood cholesterol and improve digestion.

Grapes

- Domestic crops in markets from late July, with peak time from August to November. Imported crops available from February through May.
- Good tonic for the blood; valuable cell salts build and purify the blood; improve cleansing function of the glands; strengthen liver and kidneys; diuretic properties reduce edema and urinary difficulties; acts as tonic for intestinal function; high magnesium content promotes good bowel action; iron content (darker skinned grapes) builds the blood.
- Alkaline; high in flavonoids, providing powerful antioxidant action.

Lemon and Lime

- Cooling in nature with astringent flavor and antiseptic qualities.
- Destroys putrefactive bacteria in the gut and mouth from high protein-high fat diet.
- Useful during times of cold and flu, hacking coughs, fevers and indigestion.
- High in Vitamin C, potassium and limonene (dissolves gallstones).
- Contains 5-6 percent citric acid, but has alkaline action in the body.

Lettuce

- Peak months May, June, July.
- Darker green leaves are higher in the nutrients chlorophyll, iron, Vitamin A and C.
- Acts as a diuretic; is cooling to the body.

Melons

- Alkaline; high water content.
- Deep, rich colored inner flesh high in Vitamin A, B, C and silicon

(especially when eaten close to the rind); high in minerals.

- Common varieties include: cantaloupes, honeydew (muskmelon), casaba (winter melon), watermelon.

Nectarines

- Available from June through September (imports from January through March).
- Provide potassium, carotenes, flavonoids, natural sugars; low in calories.

Okra

- An annual crop, and member of the mallow family of mucilaginous herbs.
- Alkaline; low in calories; high in natural sodium.
- Lubricates the intestinal tract and soothes irritated membranes; helps keep joints limber.

Onion

- Volatile oils give onions their flavor and "crying" factor.
- Effective in relieving cold and flu symptoms and eliminating phlegm and mucous.
- High sulfur content benefits the liver; best eaten with proteins so the sulfur can stimulate the amino acid activity to the brain and nervous system.

Parsley

- Grown year round peaking in June and July.
- Commonly used as a garnish; extremely high in nutrients.
- Alkaline; has a pungent, bitter flavor that stimulates and improves the digestion.

- High in iron, copper, chlorophyll, calcium, sodium, Vitamin C and pro-vitamin A.
- Purifies the blood; strengthens the adrenal glands; stimulates the bowels; supports kidney function.

Peach

- On the market from late May to October, the peak months are July to August.
- Alkaline; provides a cooling nature to the body.
- Builds bodily fluids; moistens lungs; relieves high blood pressure; has laxative effect.

Peas - Green

- Available from mid spring to early winter.
- Alkaline forming (fresh peas) and a rich source of incomplete protein.
- Excellent source of Vitamins A, B1, B6, C and K, manganese, folate, potassium, magnesium, iron and zinc, providing bone and heart health and energy.

Pepper - Bell

- Member of the nightshade family.
- Considered a protective food due to high content of Vitamins A, B, C and silicon (healthy hair, skin and nails); improves appetite; reduces swelling and promotes circulation.

Pineapple

- Available year round with peak months of June and July.
- Known for its bromelain content, a protein digesting enzyme which improves sluggish digestion; benefits upper respiratory tract infections; relieves overworked muscles.

- Fresh pineapple is abundant in enzymes, Vitamin C and potassium and low in calories.

Plum

- In the market from May to October, peaking in August, depending on variety.
- Known for its laxative effect and good source of Vitamin C, carotenes, flavonoids, potassium and iron.
- Acid reaction.

Radish

- Available year round with the peak season April through July.
- Pungent flavor; strong diuretic properties; stimulates digestive activity.
- Improves conditions of sinus congestion, hoarseness, phlegm, indigestion, and toxicity.
- Prevents viral infections such as the common cold or flu when eaten regularly.

Rhubarb *(see Nature's Spring Pantry in Chapter 10)*

Squash – Summer

- Low in calories; high in water content (cooling to the body).
- Excellent source of potassium, carotenes and Vitamin C
- Common varieties include: yellow (crook neck), white bush and zucchini.

Tomato

- Botanically considered a fruit; member of the nightshade family (may aggravate arthritic/inflammatory conditions).
- Peak season from June through August.

- Provides modest amounts of Vitamin C, lycopene (a carotene) and potassium.
- Healing properties tone the stomach, cleanse the liver, aid in general body detoxification and purify the blood.
- An acidic food, but after complete digestion the tomato alkalizes the blood.

Tropical Fruits

- Usually not grown in the United States (mainland) and are considered a summer fruit.
- Includes most commonly used avocado, bananas, guava, mango, papaya, and pineapple and many not-so-common exotic fruits.
- Provide a substantial source of carbohydrates, vitamins, minerals and fiber.
- With their natural sweetness, tropical fruits lend themselves to simple summer dessert dishes.

I encourage you to use wisdom when attending the ever popular, all-American backyard barbecue event. This is certainly an opportunity to be outdoors during this spectacular season and spend time with family and friends. The food offerings of this traditional gathering may be delicious, but they also hold the potential for a gastric disaster. A typical menu consists of grilled animal protein slathered in barbecue sauce, potato salad, pasta salad, baked beans, chips with a variety of dips, brownies topped with ice cream and assorted alcoholic beverages.

Now, please don't misunderstand. I am not against a delightful backyard gathering, but I urge you to use wisdom as you fill your plate. Select several items from the relish tray—remember that "pickled" foods promote a healthy gut. Also, consider choosing a fresh Summer green salad with a light vinaigrette. Grilled Summer vegetables drizzled with olive oil make a great substitute to the potato or pasta salads. A light, Summer red wine deliciously tops off the meal *and* supports healthy digestion.

Summer's fresh produce gives us great variety in tasty nutrition that supports healthy digestion and a strong heart. I hope you will enjoy these seasonal flavors and share them at your next Summer gathering.

15

Nature's Summer Recipes: Cool and Easy

The doctor of the future will give no medication, but will interest his patients in the care of the human frame, diet and in the cause and prevention of disease.
—Thomas Edison

Country Cucumber Salad (Gurke Salat)

Serves 4

In a large serving bowl, combine:

8-10 small cucumbers, washed and sliced
(with the tender peel left on)
1 small onion, sliced thinly
1 tsp. fresh dill, snipped
¼ cup sour cream
whipping cream as needed

- Thin sour cream by adding whipping cream—not whipped cream—to lightly coat the cucumber-onion mixture.
- Salt and pepper to taste. Chill before serving.

Connie's Comments: For this family favorite I choose the smaller, pickling-size cucumbers with tender outer peels. If you are using larger cucumbers, remove the tough outer peel and large seeds.

Simple Salt Cucumbers

2 small cucumbers, washed and sliced
1 Tbsp. sugar
1 tsp. Kosher salt

- In medium sized bowl, toss cucumber slices with sugar and salt.
- Cover and refrigerate for at least one hour.
- Serve cucumbers well chilled.
- These make a great side dish for Summer grilled meat and fish.

Connie's Comments: This is a surprisingly simple and delicious side dish. You'll want to double or triple the recipe for your Summer gatherings!

Three Summer Thirst Quenchers

Fruity-licious Beverage

- Add fresh cleaned fruit (blueberries, raspberries, strawberries, peaches, watermelon or cantaloupe slices) to a pitcher of purified water, green tea or sparkling water.
- Pour into a tall glass with ice and garnish with a sprig of fresh mint.

Refreshing Mint and Lime Cooler

- In a large pitcher, place a washed sliced lime and a medium sprig of fresh peppermint.
- Fill the pitcher with purified water and add ice. Pour into beverage glasses and enjoy.

Herbal "Pick-Me-Up" Beverage

- In a large pitcher, place washed fresh sprig of rosemary.
- Fill the pitcher with purified water; let the rosemary "infuse" into the water for about 1-hour before serving.
- Pour beverage into an ice-filled glass and enjoy.

Connie's Comments: This is a great afternoon beverage to naturally stimulate heart and circulation activity. Rosemary also promotes mental clarity.

Grilled Fruit

Summer grilling isn't just for meat and vegetables. Peaches, pineapple, mangos, apricots, nectarines and grapes tempt your taste buds in a whole new way when added to the grill.

- Cut washed fruit in bite size chunks or wedges, remove pits, and place on a wood or metal skewer or on a vented grilling tray.
- Prepare fruit on skewers, then lay skewers on a medium heated grill or on the top cooking rack.
- Grill for about 3 minutes or until grill marks show on fruit, then turn skewer and grill other side for 3-4 minutes until fruit is soft but not mushy.
- Remove from grill and place onto serving platter, or divide into individual servings and add a scoop of vanilla ice cream or frozen yogurt.
- Garnish with fresh sprig of mint, if desired.

Connie's Comments: Soaking wooden skewers in water before adding fruit pieces helps prevent "splinters" in the fruit when removing fruit from skewer.

Grilled Peach Salsa

Serves 4, about ¾ cup each

3-4 medium-sized ripe peaches, peeled, pitted and cut into halves
1 tsp. coconut oil
2 Tbsp. finely chopped red onion

1 small jalapeño pepper, seeded and finely chopped
1 lime, zest and juice
¼ cup fresh cilantro, finely chopped
2 Tbsp. fresh mint, finely chopped

- Preheat grill to medium. Brush cut sides of peaches with oil. Grill the peaches 3 to 5 minutes per side, until slightly softened. Let cool.
- Chop the peaches into ¼-inch pieces and place in a medium bowl. Add onion, jalapeño, lime zest and juice, cilantro and mint. Gently stir to mix completely.
- Transfer to serving bowl and serve with tortilla chips or as a topping for grilled chicken or fish.

Peachy Rice Salad

Serves 10

1-1/2 cups cooked Jasmine or Basmati rice
11 oz. whole kernel corn (frozen, cooked & drained)
  or 1-1/2 cups roasted corn cut from the cob
1 cup sliced almonds, lightly toasted
1 cup fresh peas or frozen peas, thawed
1 peach, peeled, pitted and coarsely chopped
½ cup Catalina salad dressing (see recipe below)
¼ cup chopped red onion
¼ cup chopped cilantro or fresh parsley

- Mix all ingredients in large bowl. Refrigerate until ready to serve.
- Transfer to serving bowl. Serve on bed of fresh greens if desired.

Connie's Comments: Peaches build bodily fluids, moisten the lungs, stimulate digestion and are cooling to the body. They supply a rich source of potassium, Vitamins A and C.

Homemade Catalina Salad Dressing

1/4 cup apple cider vinegar
1/3 cup mild flavored olive oil
1/2 cup ketchup
2 Tbsp. sugar
1/2 Tbsp. Worcestershire sauce
1/2 tsp. onion powder
1/2 tsp. paprika
1/2 tsp. each, sea salt and freshly ground pepper

- Place all ingredients in a shaker jar and mix well.
- Use as desired on salads, tacos and the Peachy Rice Salad recipe above.
- Refrigerate extra dressing in a covered container.

Connie's Comments: I prefer not to use commercial dressings as they usually contain canola oil, high fructose corn syrup, and an excessively high sodium content. The popular store shelf brand has 19 ingredients/additives including Red 40, Yellow 6 and Blue 1 color additives.

Summer Cherry and Quinoa Salad

Serves 6

1-1/2 cups quinoa, rinsed and drained
6 Tbsp. olive oil, divided
4 Tbsp. fresh lime juice, divided
1 bunch fresh basil
2 cups halved fresh, bing cherries
1 cucumber, peeled, seeded and diced (1-1/2 cups)
1-1/2 cups cooked chickpeas
2 large shallots, finely chopped (1/2 cup)
¼ cup sliced almonds or pine nuts
¼ cup plain low-fat yogurt

- Bring 3 cups water to a boil in pot over medium-high heat. Stir in quinoa. Reduce heat to medium-low, cover and simmer 15 minutes or until all liquid has been absorbed.
- Remove from heat and let cool, covered in pot. Transfer to serving bowl and toss with 3-Tbsp. olive oil and 2-Tbsp. lime juice. Season with salt and pepper.
- Snip fresh basil into very thin strips.
- Add basil, cherries, cucumber, chickpeas, shallots, and almonds to quinoa mixture; toss to combine. Chill 30 minutes to allow flavors to develop.
- Meanwhile whisk together yogurt, remaining 3-Tbsp. olive oil and remaining 2-Tbsp. lime juice in small bowl. Serve salad with yogurt dressing on side.

Connie's Comments: Other stone fruits (plum, nectarines, apricots) may be substituted for the cherries for flavor and color variety. Also, if you prefer, you may use fresh green peas instead of the chickpeas.

Tomato-Cucumber Summer Salad with Pita Bread

Serves 8

3-4 small cucumbers, peeled, cut lengthwise in fourths, then sliced
12 cherry tomatoes, chopped
1 small green bell pepper, seeded and finely chopped
or a small jalapeño may be used
1/2 small onion, finely chopped
2/3 cup fresh parsley, chopped
1/4 tsp. sea salt
2-4 Tbsp. fresh lemon juice
4 Tbsp. extra virgin olive oil

- Combine cucumbers, tomatoes, peppers, onion and parsley in a large mixing bowl.

- In a small mixing bowl, add lemon juice and slowly stir in oil and salt. Pour over the vegetables and gently stir thoroughly to coat.
- Chill 1 to 2 hours before serving.
- Serve with warm Pita bread.

Because of the media hype and woefully inadequate information, too many people nowadays are deathly afraid of their food, and what does fear of food do to the digestive system? I am sure that an unhappy or suspicious stomach, constricted and uneasy with worry, cannot digest properly. And if digestion is poor, the whole body in politic suffers.

~Julia Child, 1912-2004, author

16

Reflections on the Season: Savoring Summer

Summertime is always the best of what might be.
—Charles Bowden, author

Your Turn...

I invite you to take a few moments to ponder the Summers of your life, completing these thoughts to discover how you've ripened (or mellowed) through the seasons.

A favorite Summer memory with significant women in my life (mother, aunt, teacher, etc.) is:

My favorite Summer foods are:

Ideas or projects I want to see come to fruition this season are:

Summer wisdom I would share with another woman in the Summertime of her life:

The Late Summer "season" may seem fleeting, but it hints to us that a change is coming. It's time to shift, although garden foods are much the same as in the earlier Summer. But the garden is winding down for the season. I invite you to take a few relaxed moments to review the Late Summer Tree Illustration on the following page and learn the organ groups that need tending. You may find it helpful to make notes on how you'll successfully navigate this season's changes.

Late Summer

Nature's Grace Period

Stomach

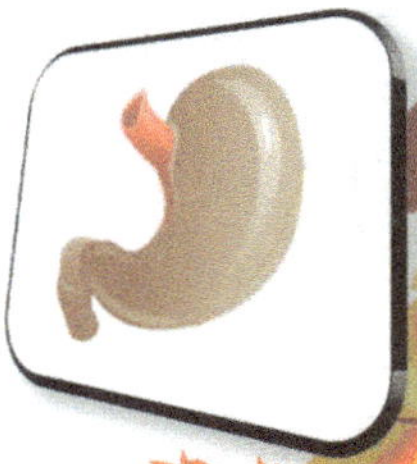

- Digestive organ in the upper-slightly left abdominal cavity that connects the esophagus to the small intestine

- Receives nourishment and prepares food for more complete digestion

Spleen

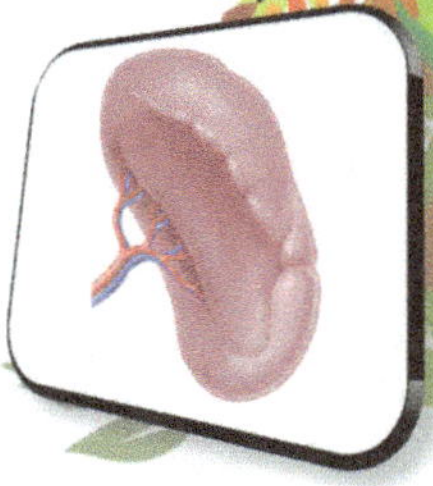

- Sac-like mass of lymphatic tissue situated near upper left of the abdominal cavity

- Forms white blood cells; filters blood and stores red blood cells; destroys and removes old or weakened red blood cells

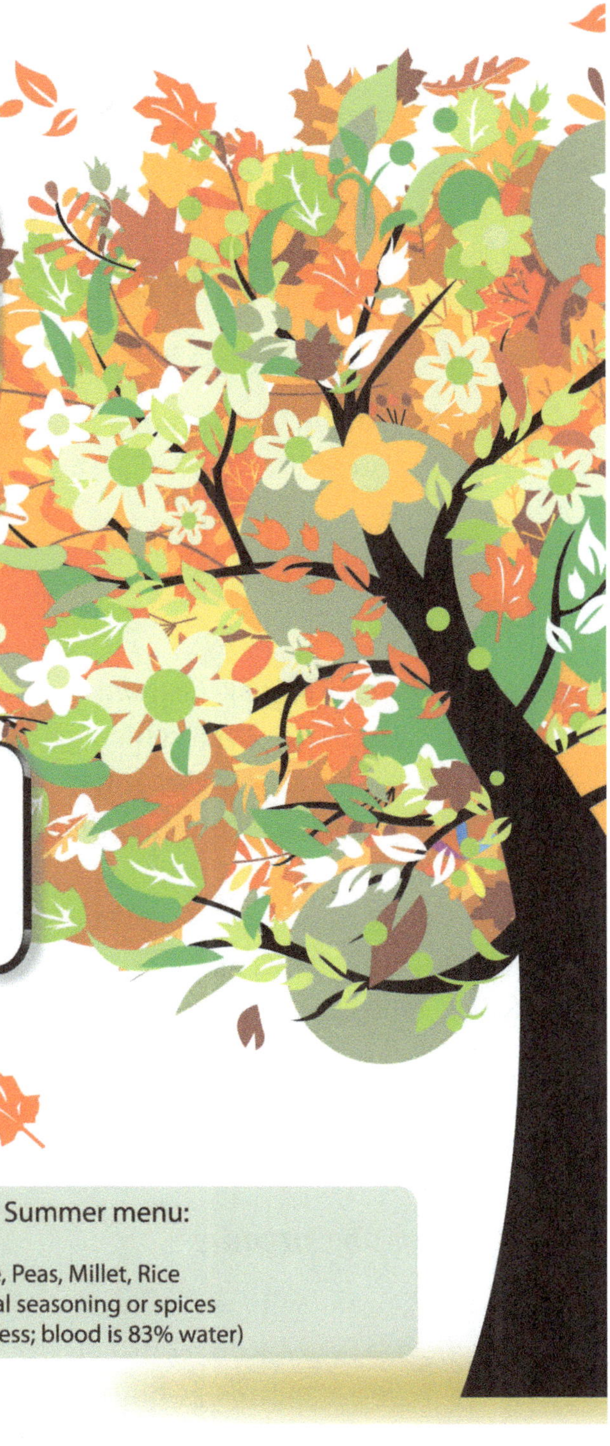

Season for change

Include these balancing foods in your Late Summer menu:

Summer Squashes, Corn, Carrots, Cabbage, Peas, Millet, Rice
Prepare simply for a mild taste; use minimal seasoning or spices
Water (hydration assists the digestive process; blood is 83% water)

17

Late Summer: A Shift from High Energy & Outward Expression

There shall be eternal summer in the grateful heart.
—Celia Thaxter, 1835-1894, American writer, poet

Getting Ready

"How much longer?" I ask. Leaning my head against the car seat, looking out the window of our 1965 robin-egg-blue Plymouth station wagon, I don't even hear the reply. My family is headed to Amarillo, Texas, a big city by my definition, on our annual Labor Day weekend school clothes shopping trip, and I feel too excited to sit still.

This means an overnight stay in the Bronco Lodge Motel and the season's final swim in a motel pool with a curved slide. We shop more this weekend than we do all year—stocking up on coats, sweaters, pleated wool skirts, knee-high socks and warm underwear. At the end of every Summer, we gratefully gather our necessities for the upcoming Fall/Autumn and Winter.

End of Season Cuttings

The season of Late Summer is that short transition following the Summer months, before Fall/Autumn officially arrives. Some years this transitional season is merely a shifting feeling in the air. At other times, it brings one last hot spell or the offering of cooler nights and crisp morning air. In whatever way Late Summer chooses to bequeath us, we know that change is coming.

This short season marks a shift from the high energy and outward expression of Spring and Summer as it draws us inward during Fall/Autumn and Winter. This is the gathering and storing season preparing us for the colder months ahead. It is time to go back to school or work. Fall/Autumn harvest will soon be brought in and fields and gardens put to rest for the Winter.

The air is perfectly quiescent and all is stillness, as if Nature, after her exertions during the Summer, were now at rest.
~John Bradbury, Scottish naturalist

In Balance for Change

Late Summer may be a short season, but it is one of intense redirection—in the natural world and within your body. This shift seems welcome to your heat-haggard body and spirit, although, you rarely are ready when the winds of change begin to blow.

The body's organs associated with this season are the stomach and spleen. Both organs contribute to the digestive process. The spleen, a sac-like mass of lymphatic tissue located near the upper left area of the abdominal cavity, distributes energy from food throughout the body. It also forms white blood cells, filters blood, stores red blood cells and destroys and removes old or weakened red blood cells. Other organs in the body depend on a healthy, fully-functioning spleen.

The stomach is positioned in the upper part of the abdominal cavity, just left and below the diaphragm. As the receiver of nourishment, it prepares food for further digestion, taking life-giving energy from food and sending it to the spleen for distribution.

Some natural healthcare professionals regard the stomach as the most sensitive organ in the body. Previously I shared information about the intricate nerve network in the small intestine. The stomach shares this finely tuned system of nerves. Have you ever experienced a nervous stomach?

Your state of mind—and emotions—are closely connected to your eating habits and how well you assimilate foods. Nourishment in the form of healthy foods and healthy experiences and relationships help keep you balanced during transitional periods.

A good digestion turneth all to health.
~George Herbert, "The Church Porch," *The Temple*-1633

Summer Solutions

At this time of year, our cellar on the farm often smelled of vinegar. Grandma began the pickling process for the last of the season cucumbers and cabbage. She layered the cucumber slices with garlic and dill, added salt water and vinegar, and then covered the large stoneware crocks with a kitchen towel. The shredded cabbage rested in the crock until it became properly fermented sauerkraut. Clean ready-to-be-filled glass jars stood in line on the cellar shelves. The flavorful food from our garden would take us into the cold Winter months, thanks to the preparations of my German grandmothers.

The diet during this transition season closely follows Summer's fresh, colorful, tasteful and nutritious choices. This is the time to savor the final flavors of the garden. Some of my clients comment that they feel unusually tired or irritable toward the end of Summer. The heat contributes in part to that fatigue, as does a heavy, high fat, high calorie diet that strains the digestive system. It's a good idea to take that siesta after a big meal so the stomach, small intestine and spleen can provide efficient digestion. When you listen to your internal rhythms and adapt appropriately, your body serves you well and energetically.

What good is the warmth of summer, without the cold of winter to give it sweetness.
~John Steinbeck, *Travels with Charley: In Search of America*

Change: You Can Count on It

This Late Summer season may be brief, but it offers much. As you awaken to the value of each season, you know how to take better care of your body. While you cannot rush into a new season before its time or command that it come sooner, neither can you linger in a past season. The seasons march on. It is not in your power to delay or speed the process. By living fully in each season, receiving its unique gifts and reciprocating with your attentive care, you promote balance on this earth and in your inner garden. Slow your pace just a bit so you feel this shift in the seasons.

The well-seasoned gardener knows this is the time to begin putting her garden to rest. Much of the high-heat produce has begun to diminish; however, many gardeners scramble to share their "zucchini-gone-wild" crop as the growing season comes to an end.

I hope you will enjoy these Late Summer recipes as you journey through this transitional season and prepare for the next season, Fall/Autumn.

18

Nature's Late Summer Recipes: Indian Summer Delights

We had gone to bed in summer, and we awoke in autumn; for summer passes into autumn in some imaginable point of time, like the turning of a leaf.
—Henry David Thoreau, 1817-1862, author of *Walden*

Spaghetti Squash – Southwest Style

Serves 4-6

1 medium sized spaghetti squash
1/4 cup diced red onion
1 clove garlic, minced
1/4 cup chicken broth
2-4 Tbsp. fresh cilantro, snipped or 2-4 tsp. dried cilantro, crushed
1/4 tsp. salt
1/4 tsp. ground cumin
1 15-ounce can black beans, rinsed
1 10-ounce can diced tomatoes with green chilies
(I use Hatch, New Mexico brand)
2 cups shredded jack cheese or a Mexican flavor cheese blend
1 avocado, sliced

- Cut the spaghetti squash in half, lengthwise; remove seeds.
- Place cut side down on baking sheet (lined with parchment paper); Cover tightly with foil.

- Bake at 350ºF. until squash is tender but not mushy, about 35-45 minutes; test for doneness by inserting fork into the center of the squash.
- In a medium skillet, on medium heat, combine chicken broth and diced onions; simmer until onions are translucent.
- Add black beans, tomatoes, garlic, cumin, cilantro, salt, and simmer until all ingredients are warmed through.
- Remove squash from oven and cool for a few minutes; using a fork, gently scrape squash in lengthwise strokes to create the "spaghetti;" discard rind.
- Place shredded squash on a platter; spoon the black bean mixture over the top; sprinkle the shredded cheese on top and garnish with avocado slices.
- Serve with a fresh green salad, blue corn chips and salsa.

Alternate ingredients you may enjoy:

Chopped red pepper may be added to the black bean mixture
Sliced black olives may be added as topping before adding cheese
A dollop of sour cream may be added on top of shredded cheese

Connie's Comments: This Late Summer hearty dish provides a high fiber, protein rich "non-meat" meal.

Simply Scrumptious Summer Squash: Have It Your Way

These tasty little treats are one of the first—and usually last—tastes of Summer. Whether you select straight-neck, crook-neck, pattypan or zucchini, these fresh from the vine, yummy little gourds won't disappoint. Pick the smaller sized squash—six to eight inches in length—to avoid the large seeds and tougher rind. These summer delights also pack a punch of potassium for heart health—along with Vitamin A, beta-carotene, lutein and zeaxanthin (for eye health)—and, of course, fiber and water!

1. Great Grillin': Cut squash into thick lengthwise slices; brush with olive oil or Italian Dressing; sear quickly on both sides; remove to serving platter and serve with fresh herb flavored butter or grated Parmesan cheese.
2. Using a mandolin, thinly slice lengthwise one yellow squash and one zucchini (cut off ends) and use in place of pasta noodles in a primavera salad or lightly stir fry using your favorite seasonings, sauce and finely grated Parmesan cheese.
3. Create a Summer slaw with grated yellow squash and zucchini; add squash to grated carrots and minced green onion and dill; toss lightly with your favorite slaw dressing. Serve and savor the flavors.
4. Cut squash into 1/4-inch chunks; place in colander and sprinkle with coarse salt; let squash sit for about 30-minutes; rinse then dry thoroughly; sauté in olive oil with minced garlic and rosemary until tender; sprinkle with grated Parmesan cheese.
5. Grated fresh zucchini adds a nutritional punch to your cookie, cake, muffin or pancake recipes. Thinly sliced zucchini can be substituted for apples in apple pie recipes.

Basic Basil Pesto

Yields 1 Cup
Prep Time: 20 Minutes

2 cups packed fresh basil leaves (2-3 bunches)
¼ cup walnut or pine nut pieces, toasted (see Tip)
¼ cup grated Parmesan or Pecorino cheese
3 Tbsp. extra virgin olive oil
2 Tbsp. water
1 large clove garlic, quartered
½ tsp. salt
½ tsp. freshly ground pepper

Tip: To toast walnuts, spread on a baking sheet and bake at 350°F., stirring occasionally until fragrant and lightly browned, 7 to 9 minutes.

- Place basil, nuts, cheese, oil, water, garlic, salt and pepper in food processor; pulse a few times, then process until fairly smooth, or to the desired consistency, scraping down the sides occasionally.
- Transfer to serving container; serve with crackers or crostini; pesto also makes a flavorful topping for grilled Summer squash.

Carrot-Apple Slaw

Serves 8

1/2 cup dried cranberries
1/2 cup fresh orange juice, divided
1 Granny Smith apple, unpeeled, cored and shredded
1 pound carrots (about 4 large), peeled and shredded
1/2 small red onion, thinly sliced
3 Tbsp. chopped fresh cilantro
1/2 cup pine nuts or walnuts (chopped), toasted
3 Tbsp. extra virgin olive oil
Freshly ground black pepper

- In a small bowl, combine dried cranberries with 1/4 cup orange juice; set aside.
- In a large bowl, toss apple with remaining 1/4 cup orange juice. Mix in carrots, red onion, cilantro and nuts.
- Drain cranberries, reserving juice. Add cranberries to apple-carrot mixture.
- Whisk together reserved orange juice and olive oil. Pour dressing over slaw. Toss well to combine and season to taste with black pepper.

Connie's Comments: This fresh produce mixture offers a delicious alternative to mayonnaise-based slaws. Bold and colorful, this dish provides a vitamin and fiber rich, heart-healthy Summer accompaniment. Pumpkin seeds may be used instead of the suggested nuts.

19

Reflections on the Season: One Last Walk in the Garden

Love is to the heart what the summer is to the farmer's year—
it brings to harvest all the loveliest flowers of the soul.
—Billy Graham, American evangelist

Your Turn...

Please take a few quiet moments to complete these thought-starters about the last days of Summer and ways to prepare for the next season.

Some ways I prepare for Summer's last days include:

This change of season makes me feel:

What I like/dislike most about the end of Summer is:

Before you read about how the Fall/Autumn season affects your physical, emotional and spiritual life, I invite you to spend a few moments looking at the Fall Tree Illustration and familiarizing yourself with the bodily organs and their functions. You will also want to review the Fall/Autumn food list as this season's dietary needs are quite different from those of the Summer season.

Fall

Gather & Celebrate the Harvest

Lungs

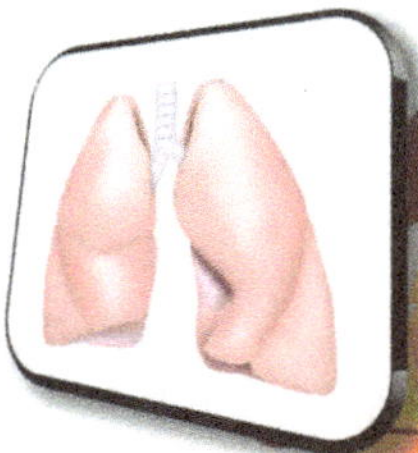

- Large cone-shaped organ with dual chambers of porous tissue

- The body's primary respiration organ and one of the body's organs of detoxification

- Transports oxygen from the atmosphere into the blood circulation and releases carbon dioxide from the blood into the atmosphere

Large Intestine

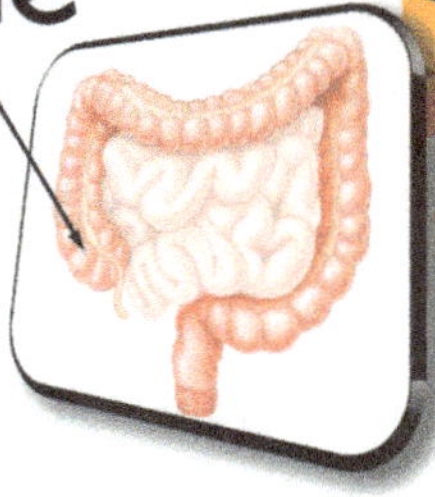

- Long tube-like organ that facilitates elimination of solid wastes from the body

- Contains numerous probiotic bacteria (healthy microflora) that promote healthy digestion and boost the immune system

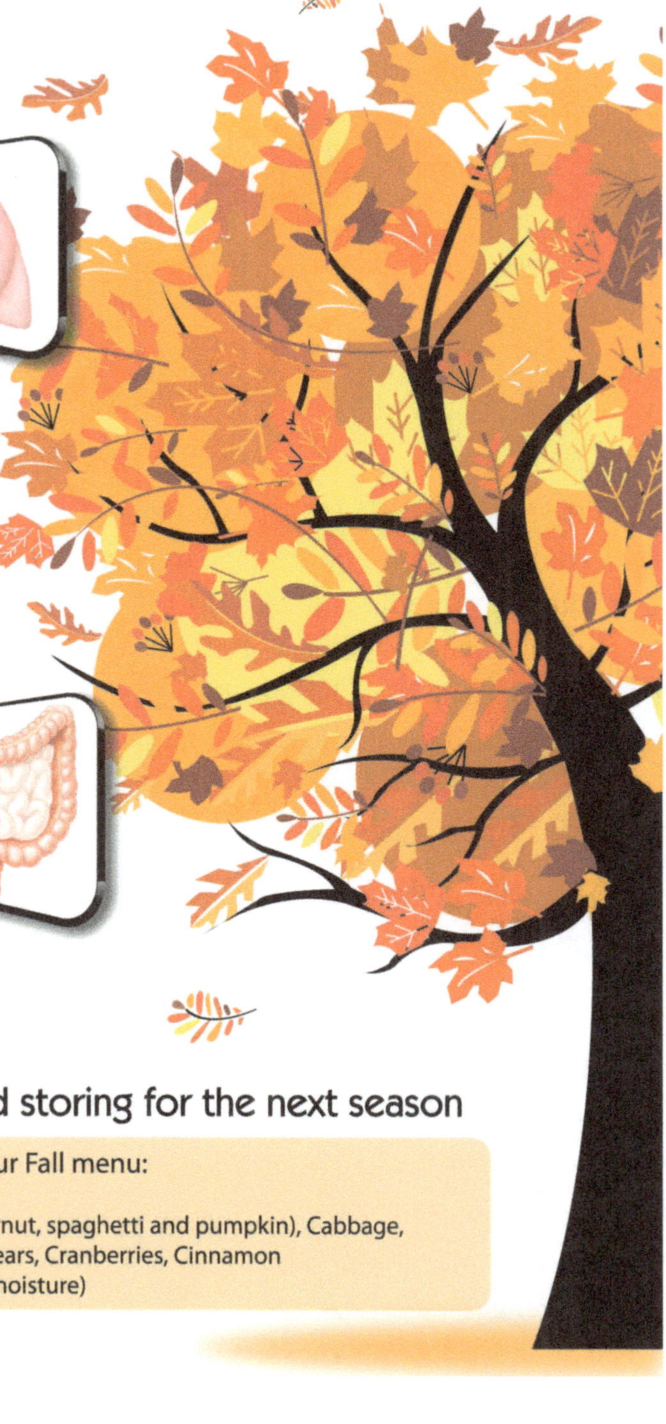

Season for preparation and storing for the next season

Include these sustaining foods in your Fall menu:

Beans, Winter squash (acorn, butternut, spaghetti and pumpkin), Cabbage,
Onions, Root vegetables, Apples, Pears, Cranberries, Cinnamon
Water (hydration maintains tissue moisture)

20

Fall/Autumn: Nature's Bountiful Gift

Every leaf speaks bliss to me, fluttering from the Autumn tree.
—Emily Bronte, 1818-1848, British novelist and poet, *Wuthering Heights*

"THE SCHOOL BUS JUST turned the corner," Mom says. She clears the breakfast dishes as my sister, Carol, and I hurry to brush our teeth and gather our school supplies. "The corner" is two miles up the road from our house but easy to see because the land in that part of Texas lies so flat. "Hurry up!" I order Carol in my bossy big sister tone. "I don't want to miss the bus."

Looking Forward to Fall/Autumn

I wanted to get back into the swing of the new school year and see my friends again after the long Summer break. It was that time of year when the school activities and changing schedules were just beginning and the farming activities were coming to a close. Dad would make preparations for one last harvest in November and then clean and store the machinery and tools until the next Spring.

Autumn (interchangeably known as fall) officially arrives around September 22nd. This exciting season brings harvests, holidays, shorter days, and crisp temperatures. Fall/Autumn reveals its fullness by splashing the trees with bold color and littering the fading lawns with fallen leaves that resemble multicolored confetti.

For me, the crackling sounds of Fall/Autumn seem to say, "Get ready. Get ready for what's ahead." Nature prepares for her long Winter's rest and teaches you and me to do the same. Fall/Autumn gives us time to gather, organize and store. It's the season to stack firewood, bring out sweaters, scarves and mittens, and fill the pantry. Come along, let's seek the season's surprises.

Autumn is a second spring when every leaf is a flower.
~Albert Camus, 1913-1960, French author and philosopher

Fall's Festive Harvest

"You girls get in the back of the truck and I'll throw these straw bales up to you," my dad says. Carol and I eagerly climb into the bed of the 1947 Chevy farm truck to help get ready for the annual church hayride. "There's room for some more," I yell, as Carol and I untie the twine and scatter the straw. Mom helps decorate the granary with scarecrows, pumpkins and straw bales draped in burlap grain sacks.

Autumn carries more gold in its hand than all the other seasons.
~Jim Bishop, 1907-1987, American journalist

Fit For Fall—Fit For Life

This season brings a noticeable change in climate, energy and diet, making it an important time to focus on your health. Historically, Fall/Autumn is a time of gathering, preparation and rest, but today's modern, highly pressurized lifestyle can create a busyness that frequently weakens your health.

The ancient Ayurvedic system of wellness embraces all aspects of your daily living, especially how the natural elements affect your health and well-being. This healing practice observes how your internal environment mirrors the external environment. For example, in the Fall/Autumn, when the air becomes dry, causing the leaves to dry and fall from their trees, you may notice that your skin feels drier and perhaps more itchy than in the Summer season. You may also experience cold hands or feet as the colder external temperatures linger in Fall/Autumn.

To help maintain balance in your body's internal rhythms through the hectic holidays and climate changes of Fall/Autumn and Winter, you may benefit from an internal cleanse early in the season. A Fall/Autumn cleanse will prepare your body for the warmer, heartier, heavier protein and fatty foods of Winter. To make this an easier process for you, I suggest you follow the simple steps I mentioned for the Spring cleanses (Chapter 9). Select fruits and vegetables from Fall/Autumn's harvest for a nutrient-rich cleanse of juices and purees. Most fruits and vegetables in this season are high in antioxidant and phytochemical plant-based nutrients that strengthen and support your immune system. This is the season to bring order back into your schedule, your plans and your health.

Commitments are like flowers in a garden:
If you over plant, none will thrive.
~author unknown

Taking In and Releasing

The lungs and large intestine are the organs influenced by the Fall/Autumn season. These two areas of the body function at their best, promoting optimal health, and long youthful life when kept clean. This pair works in tandem by providing life-giving energy from inhaled oxygen and by removing your internal trash. Attention and care given to these organs in this season may help prevent a long Winter of colds or respiratory ailments.

Clearing and Cleansing—Reaping Wellness

The large intestine (colon) deals primarily with absorbing water and nutrients, producing friendly bacteria (probiotics that assist in food digestion and vitamin synthesis), and eliminating solid wastes from the body. It measures almost six feet in length and two inches in diameter and divides into the ascending, transverse, descending and sigmoid (pelvic) colon, forming an inverted u-shaped frame around the small intestine.

This organ easily becomes over-stressed from your contemporary lifestyle and highly refined diet. Constipation, the most common digestive disorder in America, puts laxative sales near the top of the medication industry. Colon cancer affects more than 100,000 Americans yearly and almost half that number will die from the disease. These are sobering facts.

A congested large intestine contributes to several discomforts and symptoms including: headaches, head and sinus pressure, sore throats, gas (flatulence), lowered immune function and decreased energy. A backed-up colon hinders the flow of nutrients, water and life energy to the rest of the body. If prolonged, this condition may lead to more serious disorders such as Irritable Bowel Syndrome, insomnia, diverticulosis (little pouches in the colon) or colitis (inflammation of the colon).

The U. S. Department of Agriculture recommends eating 3-5 servings each of fruits and vegetables every day for sufficient dietary fiber in addition to valuable vitamins and minerals to relieve or prevent constipation. As the indigestible fiber from the fruits and vegetables passes through the large intestine, it absorbs the available water, softening and bulking the waste matter, preparing it for elimination.

Dietary fiber (also called roughage) is present in whole grains (bran), sprouted seeds, nuts, dried beans and legumes. Foods from animal sources do not contain dietary fiber, so be sure to add a couple of servings of fruits or vegetables to complete every meal.

The current Food Guide Pyramid provided by the USDA's Center for Nutrition is somewhat misleading in that it suggests 6-11 servings of grain-type foods (bread, cereal, pastries, pasta, rice) for adults. In today's food market, it is becoming more difficult for the mindful consumer to find organic, non-GMO, whole grain products. The surplus of processed grain foods (carbohydrates) is considered to be one of the contributors to the obesity factor in America today. Perhaps the American Food Guide Pyramid should be turned upside down, so that the grainy foods would be minimal and the healthy Omega fats, lean proteins, fruits and vegetables would present a more generous portion on your plate and a smaller portion around your waist!

Strong Lungs for Life

Your lungs (the body's main organ of respiration) breathe in life and disperse it throughout your entire body. Working closely with your heart and circulatory system, they take in energy as oxygen and eliminate waste in the form of carbon dioxide. Comprised of a pair of cone-shaped, spongy organs in the upper-mid-chest cavity, the lungs contain lobules, bronchi and millions of air cells. Your incredibly designed body enfolds this valuable organ with the pleura, a sac-like protection allowing for lung expansion and contraction.

The rhythm of your breath affects other rhythmic cycles in your body. Whether your breath is fast or slow, deep or shallow, erratic or rhythmic, the pace of your heart and flow of your blood circulation reflects this pattern.

Your breathing patterns reveal more about you than you may realize. When you feel anxious or driven or overly emotional, you tend to breathe more quickly and shallowly. Yet, when you breathe rhythmically and freely you usually become less affected by the unexpected changes around you and better equipped to deal with your emotions, attitudes and actions.

Do you remember the sleeping baby illustration in a previous chapter? The rhythmic, deep-from-the-diaphragm gentle breathing? As you age, your breathing often becomes shallower as you begin using only the upper chest portion of your lungs. Yoga is an excellent fitness form that teaches deep breathing exercises as a relaxation technique. The technique recommends slowing the breath and taking deep breaths when stressed, angry or afraid. This exercise calms the entire body, allowing for clarity, focus and even healing during demanding or tense-filled times.

Oxygen circulation is vital for healthy internal organs. An additional benefit of improved circulation is healthy, vibrant skin and hair. It seems wise to start taking more deep, rhythmic breaths!

Aging is not lost youth but a new stage of opportunity and strength.
~Betty Friedan, author

Understanding the Inner Fall/Autumn

Menopause, that time in a woman's life when menstrual activity naturally ceases, usually comes between the ages of 35 and 58. Some women experience a sudden end to their periods while others may be in the journey for an extended time. This season of change offers a great opportunity for women to examine their wellness style from earlier years and make alterations that fit their new health needs.

There's an abundance of well-documented, excellent information for women that provides comforting support and possible solutions for this hot-flash, night-sweat, mood-swinging season. One of my favorite resources is medical doctor, Christiane Northrup, *Women's Bodies, Women's Wisdom* and *The Wisdom of Menopause*, who consistently offers indispensable and easily accessible knowledge and wisdom for women living and even thriving through this time of change.

More scientific attention is being given to hormone health today than any other time in history. The number of medical professionals providing natural hormone therapy is increasing. This truly is a wonderful time in which to be aging—and to have the opportunity and tools to age well.

I agree with Dr. Northrup that one's food choices during this season play an important role in maintaining hormone balance. Since everything you eat alters your hormones, a diet rich in Nature's harvest provides essential nutrients for hormonal balance, weight management and emotional well-being. You help yourself by choosing to eat seasonal fruits, vegetables, nuts and seeds, as well as lean protein and restrict your intake of overly processed, manufactured foods.

All I really need is love, but a little chocolate now and then doesn't hurt.
~Lucy Van Pelt in *Peanuts*

I read several humorous books about entering and navigating this new season. I highly recommend the following titles: *Juicy Tomatoes: Plain Truths, Dumb Lies and Sisterly Advice About Life After 50,* by Susan Swartz; *Mentalpause: And Other Midlife Laughs,* by Laura Jensen Walker; and *Cooking with Hot Flashes: And Other Ways to Make Middle Age Profitable* by Martha Bolton. These female authors traveled the path before and left their wit and wisdom so that you might enjoy the journey—or at least have a laugh or two along the way. I have discovered that laughter and chocolate do make the journey more bearable. They made me more bearable, anyway!

Most women possess a keen sense of their body's messages and its internal language. (Some of us just need courage and permission to listen to our inner expressions.) This inner Fall/Autumn season offers you the opportunity and time to review who you have become and the path you want to take in the future. You have the privilege—and responsibility—to set an example of lovely, grace-filled aging for women still in their youthful seasons. I once heard someone say that aging is a natural process, but getting old is not an option. The Autumn within you prepares you to harvest the good life, so you need to plant wisely.

Every age can be enchanting, provided you live within it.
~Brigitte Bardot, actress

Living in the Light

In these shorter Fall/Autumn days, with limited natural sunlight, Seasonal Affective Disorder (SAD) affects millions of women as well as some men and children. If you notice yourself experiencing decreased energy, sweets cravings, a need for more sleep, weight gain or unusual mood changes, take note of your surroundings, habits and food choices during this time of year.

Fall/Autumn ushers in several holidays creating a smorgasbord of fun foods. These foods, usually high in calories, sugars and fats, tempt your cravings and can add extra pounds, all of which may contribute to SAD. Cooler temperatures may bring an end to outdoor exercise programs. Also, many women work in offices with no windows for natural light. Those who tend to be negatively affected by these Fall/Autumn-induced conditions would be wise to take action steps to prevent increased symptoms.

Some simple suggestions that may help chase the SAD blues away include taking a lunch break Nature walk, opening windows at home or work to let natural light shine in, maintaining a balanced natural foods diet, getting regular exercise and maintaining your sleep routine. Take a break and spend time with friends and loved ones in a relaxing, enjoyable atmosphere. Fall/Autumn offers many beautiful and bountiful surprises that can help you manage your SAD symptoms—don't miss them.
As always, if you feel severely affected, consult your wellness provider.

Snuggle In and Savor the Harvest

French fashion designer, Coco Chanel, once said, "Nature gives you the face you have at 20; it is up to you to merit the face you have at 50." Fall/Autumn offers you an exciting opportunity to look inward, to examine your journey and evaluate how you have weathered the storms so far.

I've been blessed in my life's journey to have many mother-mentor-friends. These older, wiser women taught me to explore the possibilities presented along the path and to never stop learning, dreaming and becoming. One of the many treasured lessons I've learned is that what I see on the outside is but a reflection of what I've cultivated on the inside throughout my life seasons. I believe it is important—and healthy—to love what we see.

As you prepare your Fall/Autumn menus, I encourage you to shop from Nature's Pantry frequently. These seasonal foods are truly the comfort foods your body needs and desires. You'll feel energetic and well as you navigate this season's activities.

Come forth into the light of things;
Let nature be your teacher.
~William Wordsworth, 1770-1850, English poet

21

Nature's Fall/Autumn Pantry: Abundant and Bold

Clean, tasty, real foods do not come processed in boxes or bags: they come from the earth, the sea, the field, or the farm.
—Suzanne Somers, actress

FALL/AUTUMN'S NATURAL DIET provides foods that promote efficient functioning of your lungs and large intestine. This time of the year offers the opportunity for a seasonal cleanse to prepare your body for the heavier foods of Winter. Pungent foods (garlic, onion, horseradish, ginger) offer cleansing and strengthening properties that prepare the lungs and large intestine for the coming season. This season's abundant harvest produces nutrient-dense foods that juice well, help eliminate stored toxins and strengthen this season's organs. To help you choose your Fall/Autumn meals wisely, I have prepared the following list of the season's readily available foods.

Apple

- Available year round, in numerous varieties.
- Alkaline; provides pectin (fiber that binds and eliminates toxins from the intestinal tract); helps produce bodily fluids (moisture) and protects lungs from cigarette smoke.

Carrot

- Grown year round.
- Alkaline; sweet in flavor with bitter tops (greens may be snipped into soups, salads or broth stock).
- High content beta-carotene (pro-vitamin A) an antioxidant that promotes eye health and protects against cancer.
- Stimulates elimination and strengthens the lungs.

Celery

- Available year round with peak months from November through May.
- Alkaline; high in natural sodium and silicon (the "youth" maintainer).
- Helps balance high protein meals—good in chicken or tuna salad.

Cranberry

- On the market from September until March, with peak months of October through December.
- Highly acidic; used more often for medicinal properties than nutritional value; mostly used for urinary tract infections.
- Most commercial juices are only 1/3 pure juice mixed with water and sugar.

Cruciferous Group

- Includes broccoli, Brussels sprouts, cabbage, cauliflower, collard greens, cress, horseradish, kale, kohlrabi, mustard, radish, rutabaga, turnip.
- Most are frost tolerant, making a longer growing season.
- High sulfur content (gas forming) aids the circulation, which keeps the body warm in colder climates.

- High in components that increase antioxidant defense mechanisms and anti-cancer properties.

Date

- Available from September until May, with November the peak month.
- Excellent source of natural sugar, much healthier than refined sugar.
- Heat producing in the body, providing a good source of energy for cold weather.

Fig

- On the market from June until November, peaking in September and October.
- High natural sugar content; great energy food for cold climates.
- High in potassium, calcium, magnesium, iron, copper and manganese.
- Alkaline; helps balance highly acidic diet of meat and fats; nourishes and tones the intestinal tract.

Grape

- Domestic crops on the market from late July until March, with peak months of August through November; the emperor grape is usually available in October and is a Thanksgiving and Christmas favorite.
- Alkaline; high magnesium and water content benefits sluggish bowels.

Jerusalem Artichoke

- A member of the sunflower family, it is not related to the globe artichoke.
- Sweet flavor; nourishing to the lungs; supports "healthy" bacteria in the intestinal tract; relieves constipation.
- Beneficial to diabetics, having specific polysaccharides that improve blood sugar balance.

Jicama (HEE-ka-ma)

- A turnip shaped root vegetable high in water content; used in raw vegetable juices, salads or vegetable trays.
- High potassium content (electrolyte aiding in maintenance of water balance and distribution, acid-alkaline balance, muscle, nerve and heart function).

Onion

- Volatile sulfurous oil gives onion its distinctive odor, flavor and "crying" factor.
- Pungent quality contributes to healing ability, especially for lung conditions.
- Clinical studies show onions help lower cholesterol levels in the blood; prevent formation of blood clots; lower blood pressure and promote warmth in the body (increasing circulation and energy).
- High in the anti-cancer bioflavonoid, quercetin.
- Varieties include: chives, leek, onion, scallion, shallot.

Pear

- Many varieties; the Bartlett is most popular, thriving in cool summers and mild winters.

- Excellent source of water soluble fiber, including pectin (pears contain more pectin than apples), a fiber that helps tone intestines, moisten lungs and lower cholesterol.
- Good energy food in colder weather, especially if eaten as a dried fruit.

Pepper

- Member of the nightshade family (with eggplant, potatoes, tomatoes).
- Good source of Vitamin C, especially when eaten raw.
- Capsaicin, the compound making peppers hot, acts as a pain reliever and is used in many topical formulas for muscle aches.
- Eating hot peppers speeds the metabolism, increases circulation, opens sinuses and breaks up mucous in the lungs.

Pomegranate

- Latin word meaning "apple with many seeds".
- Growth season is September through December with October its peak month.
- The juice is very tart, making it an excellent tonic for the bladder and kidneys.
- Phytonutrients help decrease damage from LDL cholesterol, lower arterial plaque and balance blood pressure.

Potato

- Member of the nightshade family (with peppers, eggplant, tomatoes).
- Most modern varieties are available year round.
- Mild, slightly sweet flavor; the outer skin being higher in nutrients than the center flesh (nearly 60 percent of the potassium content is in the peeling).

- Provides Vitamin C, enzymes and minerals; acts as a diuretic and lubricant to intestines.

Potato – Sweet

- Not related to the common potato.
- Rich in carotenes, Vitamin C, calcium, and potassium.
- Helpful in removing toxins from the body; strengthens the elimination system.

Squash – Winter

- Member of the gourd or melon family, these thick skinned squash include: acorn, butternut, delicata, Hubbard, kabocha and pumpkin.
- Winter squash are a nutrient dense food in their peak from October through December and store well through the Winter months.
- Provides high amount of carotenes, complex carbohydrates, potassium and several B-vitamins supporting the body against many cancers.

Nuts – Seeds – Whole Grains

Seeds have all the chemical elements, nutrients and nucleic acids to produce new life.
~Dr. Bernard Jensen, *Foods That Heal: A Guide Understanding and Using the Healing Power of Natural Foods*, 1988

- Abundant in the Late Summer and Fall/Autumn harvest; very concentrated food form; heat producing for energy.

- Contain greatest amount of essential fatty acids of all unprocessed foods; best source of Vitamin E.
- High in vitamins, minerals, amino acids, carbohydrates and essential fats.

Almond

- Available year round, with peak freshness in mid-Summer; a cousin of the peach, apricot and cherry tree (hard seeds or pits).
- Sweet flavor, often called "King of Nuts" because of abundant nutrient value.
- High in potassium, magnesium, phosphorus, protein and monounsaturated fats.

Pecan

- Available year round with harvest season from September through December, depending on part of the country grown.
- High in antioxidants, unsaturated fats (kernel is 65-70 percent oil) and protein.
- Provides over 19 vitamins and minerals including Vitamins A and E, folic acid, calcium, magnesium, phosphorus, potassium, several B-vitamins, and zinc.

Walnut

- Available year round with harvest in December; considered "brain food" (the appearance of the walnut resembles the human brain).
- Excellent source of omega-3 essential fatty acids (helps cognitive function); high antioxidant activity; easily usable form of melatonin; high in manganese and copper.

Flax Seed

- Available year round in several varieties as whole or ground seeds, with harvest from late September through early October.
- Light nutty flavor provides rich supply of alpha linolenic acid (an omega-3 fat), fiber, magnesium, manganese, phosphorous, folate and copper.
- Benefits include: reduced inflammatory conditions (asthma, arthritis, migraine headaches and osteoporosis) and laxative effect for congested colon.

Pumpkin Seeds

- Available year round but freshest during the Fall/Autumn pumpkin season.
- Also known as "pepitas," they are high in the minerals magnesium, manganese, phosphorous, iron, copper, and zinc.
- Benefits include: bone health, prostate protection, lowered cholesterol, anti-inflammatory agents and colon/spleen-pancreas support.

Sesame Seeds

- Available year round but harvested by October, before frost.
- Very good source of manganese, copper, calcium, magnesium, iron, phosphorous, Vitamin B1, zinc and fiber.
- Nutrients help prevent PMS and migraine headaches, relieve rheumatoid arthritis and respiratory inflammation and improve bone health.

Sunflower Seeds

- Available year round, with domestic harvest from late August through early October, depending on locale.

- The mild nutty flavor is loaded with health benefits including Vitamin E (antioxidant that neutralizes free radical damage), magnesium, selenium, phosphorous folate and about 25 percent protein.
- Helpful in lowering cholesterol, calming nerves and muscles, curbing hunger, enhancing energy and correcting constipation.

Amaranth

- A warm weather crop dating back to the ancient Aztecs and harvested the end of July up to Labor Day.
- Excellent source of protein (almost ideal amino acid balance), calcium and Vitamin C.
- Used in breads, cakes, soups, grain dishes, or cooked as a hot cereal.

Millet

- Drought resistant crop harvested about September.
- Alkaline, gluten-free and easy to digest; high in quality protein, B-vitamins and silicon (the "beautifying" mineral that strengthens connective tissue and bone, promotes healthy hair, skin and nails).
- Supports the stomach, spleen and pancreas, relieves indigestion and is anti-fungal.

Quinoa (pronounced "keen-wa")

- A cool weather crop with similar properties of amaranth.
- Considered a "super grain" for its nutritional values including complete protein, potassium, magnesium, zinc, copper, manganese and the B-vitamins.
- Cooked like rice, it may be eaten as a hot cereal or pilaf or cold in a salad or added to smoothies.

Connie's Comments: Many grains including wheat, barley, oats and rye are available during the Fall/Autumn season. When they are purchased and eaten as "close to nature" as possible, they retain a higher nutrient content. Perhaps this list highlights seeds and grains that may be unfamiliar to you. Be bold—experiment with something new. Also, be a savvy shopper and ask where and how the seeds and grains are grown.

Spices to Warm and Heal

The fresh herbs that greeted you in the Spring and Summer may be familiar to you as dried, ground spices to pep up the flavor of your dishes in the colder seasons. The earliest Native Americans and ancient Aztecs among others regarded spices as a critical food-medicine that were traded—and pirated—because they improved the quality, and very often the longevity of life.

The nutritional properties of spices remain much the same as the fresh-picked version with these considerations:

- Some nutrient values or flavor elements may be reduced in the drying process and extended storage.
- Many dried spices retain high ORAC levels (Oxygen Radical Absorbance Capacity) which measure the antioxidant potential of the plant.

I hope you will consider this short and simple list of spice cabinet remedies for your Fall/Autumn and Winter recipes.

A man may esteem himself happy when that which is his food is also his medicine.
~Henry David Thoreau, 1817-1862, American naturalist and author

Cayenne

- This warming spice stimulates circulation thereby improving heart, artery and capillary function; mixed with water a pinch of cayenne makes an effective gargle for a sore throat.
- The flavor packs a punch of "zesty-hot" to any dish especially Southwestern or Mexican cooking.

Cinnamon

- This aromatic and fragrant spice comes from the bark of Cinnamomum trees native to South America, Southeast Asia and the Caribbean; the drying process produces the tubular rolls or "cinnamon sticks".
- Recorded use dates to ancient Egypt, 2000 BC, for treatment of sore throats, coughing, and arthritic conditions.
- Health promoting properties include exceptionally high antioxidants; increased digestive enzyme secretions; improved blood sugar and lipid levels; reduced bacterial and fungal infections.
- Known throughout the world as a flavoring for dishes ranging from main courses to condiments and sauces to desserts; extreme amounts may cause respiratory distress or inflammation.

Cumin

- The seeds provide an excellent source of iron, manganese, calcium, magnesium phosphorus, selenium, zinc, B-complex vitamins, Vitamins A, C, E and dietary fiber; seeds may be steeped as a tea or ground as a spice.
- Historically used medicinally to improve energy and immune function; for digestive support (enzyme production); powerful free radical scavenging properties.
- Adds a nutty peppery flavor to chili, Mexican dishes and Indian and Middle Eastern curries.

Ginger

- The root (rhizome) of this aromatic plant is used in medicinals and culinary creations; it may be used fresh, dried, powdered or ground, or as an oil (essential oil).
- Commonly used (fresh) as a digestive aid to stimulate production of saliva and bile, relieve gastrointestinal distress, and calm nausea from morning sickness to motion sickness; relieves joint discomforts and headaches.
- Long history in Chinese cooking as well as in condiments and curries of Southeast Asia.
- Well-known ingredient in gingerbread and ginger ale.

Paprika

- This vibrant red powder comes from capsicum peppers (dried and finely ground).
- Loaded with nutrients, including: Vitamins A, C, E, iron (blood builder) and carotenoids (pigments giving the deep red coloring) for added health benefits.
- Historically used medicinally as an anti-bacterial, anti-inflammatory, external pain reliever, digestion stimulant (enzyme production) and circulatory system support.
- Frequently blended with garlic and other spices and used as a rub for chicken, fish, pork or lean beef.
- May be added to hummus, soups or egg dishes for additional color, flavor and health benefits.
- An excellent resource for purchasing paprika and recipes: *For the Love of Paprika* by John Czingula at *PaprikaRocks.com.*

Sage

- A sister herb to rosemary, and member of the mint family, is high in antioxidant, anti-inflammatory properties and volatile oils which help prevent cellular oxidation (free radical damage).

- Long regarded as an excellent memory enhancer.
- Early Greeks and Romans used sage as a meat preservative; it pairs well with poultry and pork.
- Sage lends a strong, often over-powering flavoring, so use sparingly as an addition to baked breads, mild cheeses, stuffing, and pasta dishes.

Turmeric

- A cousin to ginger, and a member of the Zingiberaceae family, this spice is made from the root of the Curcuma longa plant.
- Used in culinary, medicinal and esthetic purposes, this spice offers antioxidant, anti-bacterial and anti-inflammatory properties.
- An excellent source of manganese, iron, Vitamin B6, copper, potassium and fiber.
- One of the most researched plant foods showing promise for cardiovascular protection, improved liver-gall bladder function, inflammatory bowel disorders, lowering cholesterol and brain function protection.
- Best known for its use in curries, egg dishes, rice and lentils.

Connie's Comments: This short list of my favorite Fall/Autumn and Winter spices not only complement the flavor of food, but promote health during these colder months. Please consult with a professional nutritionist if you are seeking therapeutic support.

Old gardeners never die, they just run out of thyme.
~Garden saying

22

Nature's Fall/Autumn Recipes: A Hearty and Healthy Harvest

Live each season as it passes, breathe the air, drink the drink, taste the fruit and resign yourself to the influences of each.
—Henry David Thoreau, 1817-1862, author

Millet Fruit Balls

1 cup cooked millet (follow package cooking instructions)
½ cup pecans, finely chopped
½ cup almonds, finely chopped
½ cup raisins or dried cranberries or dried currants, finely chopped
½ cup dried apple, finely chopped
½ cup dried apricots, finely chopped
1 Tbsp. fresh squeezed orange juice

- Mix all ingredients in a food processor or mix the above ingredients by hand.
- Form small balls, about the size of a whole in-shell walnut.
- Roll in chopped nuts or organic coconut flakes.
- This makes a healthy candy or dessert choice and travels well for sack lunches.

Stuffed Acorn Squash

Serves 4

2 cups cooked quinoa or wild rice (follow package cooking instructions)
2 medium acorn squash cut in half from stem end to point, remove seeds
½ cup walnuts or pecans, toasted then chopped
½ cup dried cherries or cranberries
¼ tsp. ground cinnamon
Extra virgin olive oil or sesame oil
Grated Romano or Parmesan cheese, optional

- Preheat oven to 350°F.
- Brush a light coating of oil on the cut surfaces of squash.
- Mix the remaining ingredients, divide and stuff each squash with the mixture.
- Place squash halves in baking dish, cover and bake for 45 minutes or until squash is tender but not mushy.
- Remove from oven, sprinkle grated cheese on top if desired, then transfer to serving platter.

Basic Pumpkin Soup

Serves 4

2 cups cooked fresh pumpkin or one 15-ounce can pumpkin puree (not pumpkin pie mix)
3 cups organic chicken broth
1 medium onion, finely chopped
2-3 medium cloves garlic, finely minced
1 Tbsp. extra virgin olive oil

- Sauté onion and garlic in oil in a large stock pot until soft.

- Pour half the pumpkin puree and half the broth into a blender, blend until smooth, and then add to stock pot.
- Repeat the process with the remaining broth and pumpkin.
- Cook on medium heat until soup gently bubbles ... for thinner soup, add more broth.
- Pour into serving bowls and top with toasted pumpkin seeds.

Connie's Comments: For variations on this basic soup, you may add cooked black beans, corn and roasted red peppers for a hearty stew. Herbs and spices such as dill, cilantro, cumin, curry or cayenne promote flavor-with-flair to your Fall/Autumn soup recipes.

One cannot think well, love well, sleep well if one has not dined well.
~Virginia Woolf, 1882-1941, English novelist

Roasted Autumn Vegetables

Serves 6

4 pounds assorted root and seasonal vegetables, washed, peeled and cut in bite-size cubes. Select from: fingerling potatoes, carrots, rutabagas, parsnips, golden beets, Brussels sprouts, celery, onion, garlic, turnips, sweet potato or butternut squash.
1/2 cup olive oil
1-1/2 Tbsp. Herbs de Provence with Lavender (recipe below)

- Preheat oven to 400°F.
- In very large mixing bowl, add vegetables and toss to coat with oil.
- Transfer vegetables to a large baking dish or roasting pan (or two smaller baking dishes) and sprinkle with Herbs de Provence. Cover baking dish(s) with foil. Place in oven.

- Bake for 45-minutes, then remove foil and gently toss vegetables. Return to oven without foil covering for another 15-20 minutes or until vegetables are tender but not mushy.
- Transfer to serving platter.

Herbs de Provence

3 Tbsp. dried oregano leaves
3 Tbsp. dried thyme leaves
1 tsp. dried basil leaves
1 tsp. dried sage leaf
3 Tbsp. dried savory
2 Tbsp. dried lavender flowers
1 tsp.dried rosemary

- Combine and mix well.
- Store the mixture in small airtight jar in a cool dark location.

Kahlua Candied Yams

Serves 6

4 medium-size yams or sweet potatoes, scrubbed, peeled and cut into 1/2" rounds
1/4 cup butter, melted
1/4 cup brown sugar or substitute
1/2 cup Kahlua
1/4 cup heavy whipping cream or half-and-half

- Preheat oven to 350°F.
- Place cut yam rounds closely together in large glass baking dish.
- In heavy skillet, on medium-low heat, melt butter with the sugar; add Kahlua and cream; stir until sugar has dissolved.

- Pour Kahlua mixture over yams; cover with foil. Bake for about 1-hour or until yams are fork tender and liquid is bubbly. Check at 45-minutes for doneness.
- Chopped pecans may be added for a topping, if desired.

Connie's Comments: I do my best to keep added sugars to a minimum. You may use a natural sweetener such as coconut sugar or xylitol, as they are a 1:1 exchange with sugar.

Sweet Potato Rounds

Serves 8

6 Tbsp. olive oil, divided
6 large sweet potatoes, scrubbed, peeled, cut into 3/4" rounds
3/4 cup toasted and cooled pecan halves, chopped
1 large shallot, minced
4 stalks celery, finely chopped
10 sprigs flat-leaf parsley, finely chopped
2 Tbsp. dried cranberries or cherries, minced
3 oz. medium-to-firm goat cheese, crumbled
4 tsp. red wine vinegar
1 tsp. smooth Dijon mustard
Salt and pepper (freshly ground)

- Preheat oven to 400°F.
- Prepare large baking sheet with generous olive oil coating (about 1-2 Tbsp.); parchment paper may also be used to line the baking sheet, omitting the olive oil coating.
- Place sweet potato rounds on sheet in single layer. Sprinkle with salt and pepper.
- Roast for 10-15 minutes then carefully turn each round to roast top side for another 10-12 minutes. Underside should be blistery, puffy and browned and should release easily from baking sheet

with a spatula; continue roasting until top side is browned like the underside; prepare topping while potato rounds are in the oven.

- In large bowl combine pecans, shallots, celery, parsley, cranberries and goat cheese.
- In a small bowl whisk together 4-Tbsp. olive oil, vinegar and mustard; pour half over the topping mixture and toss until well blended.
- Remove roasted potato rounds from oven (they should be fork-tender in center); arrange on serving platter; scoop a spoonful of topping mixture on top of each potato round.
- Drizzle remaining dressing over the top to taste.
- Serve immediately.

Connie's Comments: I love this variation of the traditional sweet potato recipes. This is the perfect addition to my Thanksgiving-Christmas-New Year's dinner menu. My family loves to nibble through the holiday season, so these Sweet Potato Rounds make a delicious, filling and healthy appetizer.

Autumn Roots Au Gratin

Serves 8

About 1-pound of each root vegetable; washed, peeled and thinly sliced (a mandolin makes slicing these firm roots much easier):
Yellow or Red Beets
Sweet potato or Yam
Parsnips (slice lengthwise and remove woody inner core before slicing thinly to bake)
Rutabaga or Turnip
3 Tbsp. Extra virgin olive oil, divided
1 cup thinly sliced shallots

1-1/3 cups whole milk, divided
3 Tbsp. all-purpose flour
1-1/2 cups finely shredded Gruyere cheese or shredded Parmesan and Romano if preferred, divided
1 Tbsp. chopped fresh thyme or 1 tsp. dried
1/2 tsp. salt
1/4 tsp. freshly ground pepper
1 cup lightly toasted whole wheat breadcrumbs or panko (Japanese bread crumbs)

- Preheat oven to 375°F.
- Coat a 9x13-inch baking dish with butter or olive oil.
- In a medium saucepan, heat 2-tablespoons of olive oil over medium heat; add shallots, stirring constantly until lightly browned, about 3-4 minutes; add 1-cup milk and bring to a simmer.
- In a small bowl, combine flour and remaining 1/3-cup of milk; whisk briskly to make a smooth paste; stir into the hot milk mixture and continue whisking until the sauce thickens and begins to bubble, 1-2 minutes.
- Remove sauce from the heat; stir in 3/4-cup of cheese, thyme, salt and pepper.
- Combine remaining cheese and 1-Tbsp. olive oil in a small bowl.
- Layer the vegetable slices in the baking dish; drizzle the cheese sauce over the top, then sprinkle with breadcrumb mixture.
- Cover with foil and bake the gratin for 1-hour, until vegetables are almost fork tender; uncover and bake until it is bubbling and the top is lightly golden. Let cool for about 15-minutes before serving.

Connie's Comments: This warming, baked dish uses the last pick of Fall/Autumn's harvest. Select your favorite root vegetables, but remember, red beets will leave their deep color throughout the layers.

Golden Milk with Turmeric

Serves 2

2 cups canned coconut milk
1/2 cup purified water
1 tsp. powdered Turmeric spice
1 tsp. ground cinnamon
1 tsp. raw (local) honey or maple syrup
1/2 tsp. ground ginger
a pinch of freshly ground black pepper

- In a 1-qt. saucepan over low-medium heat, bring all ingredients almost to a boil.
- Stir continuously to infuse flavors and prevent scorching, about 3-5 minutes.
- Let mixture sit for a few minutes, then pour into a cup and enjoy.

Connie's Comments: You may want to use 1-tablespoon each of freshly grated ginger and turmeric root instead of the powdered spice. Blending all ingredients on high in your blender makes a smoother Golden Milk. For additional health benefits, you may choose to add one teaspoon organic coconut oil and a pinch of cayenne powder. The ground black pepper increases the absorption of nutrients.

This is a wonderful cold-and-flu beverage with hundreds of immune-boosting health benefits. Taken before bed, it promotes relaxation. This spice is called the "spice of life" in India.

23

Reflections on the Season: Gathering and Storing for Fall/Autumn

It's fun to get together and have something good to eat at least once a day. That's what human life is all about—enjoying things.
—Julia Child, 1912-2004, author of *Mastering the Art of French Cooking*

Your Turn...

I invite you to take a few moments to complete these Fall/Autumn thought-starters. As you respond, ponder the different ways you have been influenced by the Fall/Autumn experiences in your life.

Fall/Autumn makes me feel:

Seasonal goodies I love to stock up on include:

My favorite Fall/Autumn activity is:

I enjoy gathering with friends or family for:

Special Fall/Autumn rituals or traditions I like include:

Winter is coming. Your pantry is stocked from the produce of the season. The Winter Tree Illustration that follows may appear bare and hint of inactivity. However, be assured that there are many life-preserving activities going on beneath the surface. Your body requires seasonal care during the Winter months. As you review the illustrated Winter Tree on the next page, think about the ways you might achieve your desired health traits and avoid the "bugs" that can bring you down during this season.

Winter

Season for Inner Nourishment and Rest

Kidneys

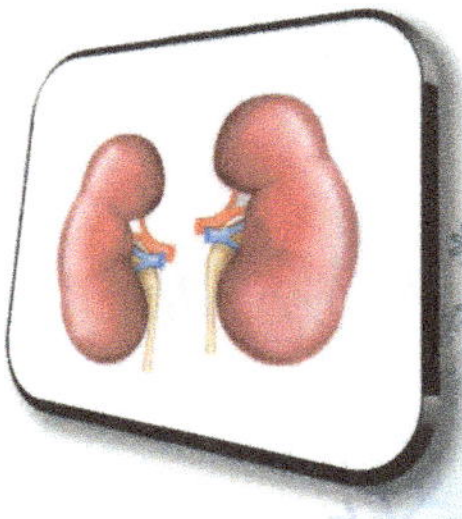

- Organ pair that circulates body's water

- Filters blood through the bladder and eliminates urine

- Maintains body's acid/alkaline balance

Bladder

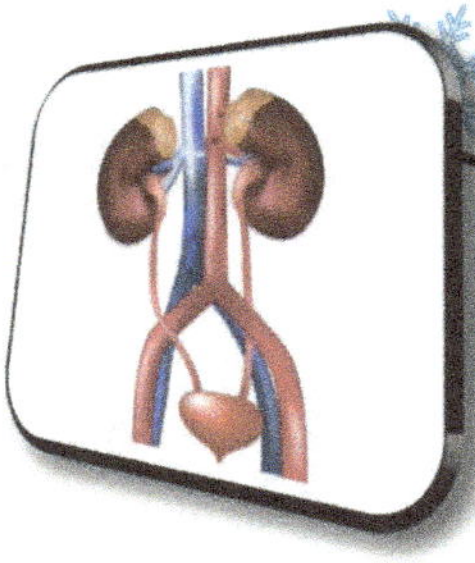

- A thick muscular pear-shaped organ in the pelvic region attached to the kidneys by two long thin tubes called ureters

- The holding/storage sac for urine from the kidneys until it is ready to be eliminated; a healthy adult bladder can hold up to 16-ounces of urine comfortably for 2-5 hours

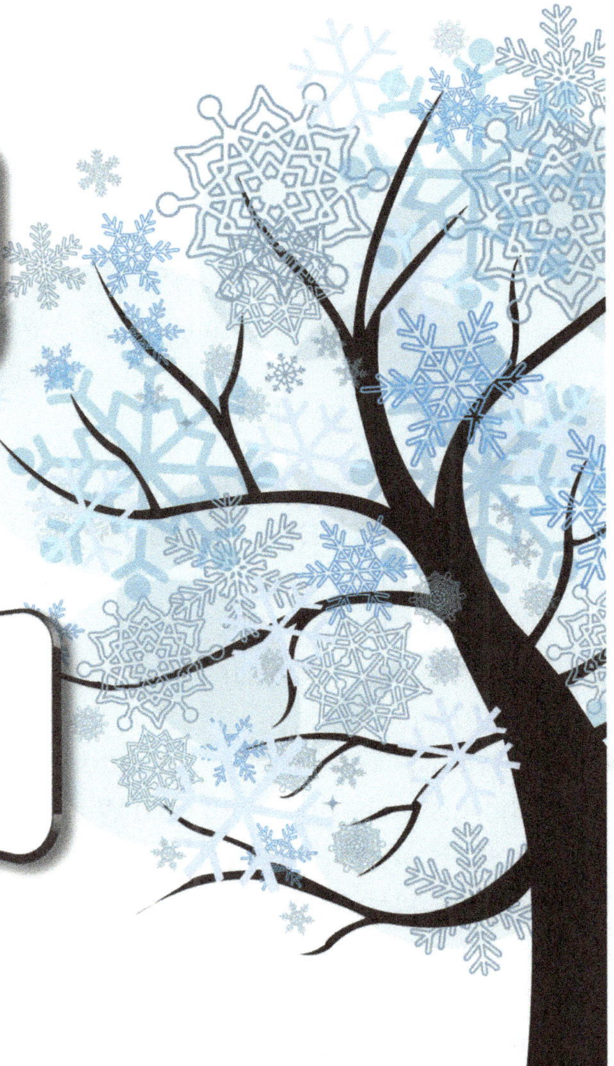

Season for Warmth and Rest

Include these warming foods in your Winter menu:

Whole grains, nuts, seeds, Root vegetables, Apples,
Pears, Dates, Cranberries, Cinnamon
Water (hydration is critical to proper function of kidneys and bladder)

24

Winter: Nature at Rest

Snowflakes are one of nature's most fragile things, but just look what they can do when they stick together.
—Vesta M. Kelly, writer

"DID YOU PUT THE dogs in the barn?" Mom asks. As the winds blow stronger and the sky darkens, she continues, "Did you leave anything lying around outside?"

"Carol put the dogs in and I checked the yard. Everything's put away, Mom," I answer.

I watch as Dad checks the batteries in our flashlights and transistor radio, just as he does with each Winter storm. Once safely inside the house, I stare out the fogged kitchen window as the snow flies fiercely in the howling wind. Soon the drifts accumulate and drape gracefully along the fence rows and roof tops like heavy frosting on a cake. During Nature's snowy blast, I feel safe and warm indoors—ready for all that this Winter season is sure to bring. Although the garden and fields won't require our constant attention until next spring, we know our animals will need us to feed them in the morning—snow or no snow.

As a young girl, I liked Winter because my family spent more time together indoors. We played the piano and sang or watched movies and ate popcorn (long before Netflix and microwave ovens). Our house was small, so we weren't scattered about. Carol and I played with our Barbie dolls and read Nancy Drew mystery books. Dad read the *Progressive Farmer* magazine and planned his Spring farming while Mom cleaned, organized, cooked and took care of us.

Glow with the Season

Winter makes its appearance on December 21st and lingers until around late March or sometimes longer in various parts of the country. Longer nights and shorter days beckon us indoors for warmth, nourishment and protection. In order to be protected and nourished until sprouting time in Spring, Nature sends her energy deep into the earth. This season brings much needed rest and regeneration for both the soil and the body. It's a time to reflect on the past and anticipate the future. Nature's landscape reveals a bareness unknown to the other seasons. Winter touches our senses in many curious ways. Bundle up; it's Winter.

I prefer winter and fall, when you feel the bone structure in the landscape—the loneliness of it—the dead feeling of winter. Something waits beneath it—the whole story doesn't show.

~Andrew Wyeth, 20th century painter

Winter's Wonder: A Simple Season

In Winter it may feel harsh to view nature stripped of her colorful foliage and fruit from previous seasons. Yet bare branches reaching out like boney fingers, fallow ground waiting for the first snow, and a monotone earth and sky declare simplicity at its finest. This season encourages you to adopt a simpler style as well. In his book, *Lightposts for Living: The Art of Choosing a Joyful Lif*e, Thomas Kinkade writes, "True simplicity begins when you learn to enjoy the amazing abundance of what is already yours." Some women do not favor the Winter season so they spend energy complaining rather than enjoying its unique qualities and health opportunities. Maybe it is time for you to explore the merit of Winter's characteristics and gifts.

Although the true Winter season suggests a quieter, restful, comfort-and-joy time, most calendars groan under the load of seasonal and holiday activities. Contemporary technology and progress sometimes takes you farther from the simple basics of Nature's rhythms. I've already mentioned the adverse affects of chronic busyness on your overall health and vitality. Several of my clients suffer frequent—but often unnecessary—illness, pain and emotional upheaval during the Winter. Pain, restlessness or distress often indicate that it is time to make some lifestyle changes—physically, intellectually, emotionally, and spiritually—for optimum wellness.

In winter, a voice says: "Be gentle, slow down, let your soul catch up with your body."
~Verna Patrick, quoted from *Health Wisdom for Women*, January 1998

Winter Harmony for Lifelong Balance

Valuable health lessons come with Winter's gifts. Spring, Summer and Fall/Autumn provide activity, growth, excitement, and long busy days often ending in exhaustion. Winter offers a respite from high energy to rest and regeneration—a time to germinate and prepare for Spring's renewal. Living in harmony with Winter means balancing incoming and outgoing energy in all areas—activity, food, rest, and emotions. Attention to this can promote well-balanced health throughout your life.

To be interested in the changing seasons is a happier state of mind than to be hopelessly in love with spring.
~George Santayana, philosopher, poet and novelist

Usually the holiday spirit and schedule begins around the Fall/Autumn harvest and continues energetically through the Winter months. Because of this, Winter is a good season to practice extreme health care. Winter brings a special time of family traditions and seasonal celebrations that usually center on plenty of food and activity. Learning to care for the body's organs that are influenced by the Winter season can bring you closer to living in balance during all the seasons.

As you noticed while reviewing the Winter Tree Illustration, your kidneys and bladder (along with the urethra and a pair of ureters) are the internal organs associated with the Winter months. These organs make up the urinary system and play an important role in the body's ability to excrete wastes. Water is an essential fluid in the human body through which all things pass. Blood circulation, lymphatic flow, saliva, perspiration, tears, urine and sexual fluids depend on adequate internal hydration. The kidneys and bladder are vital to this filtering process.

Unpretentious but Not Unimportant

The kidneys, a pair of purplish-brown bean shaped (that would be kidney bean shaped) organs, sit at the back of the abdominal cavity on either side of the spinal column.

They are securely supported and protected in a mass of fat and held in place by layers of connective tissue. These fist-sized organs rest above the waistline rather than in the small of the back, as many believe. The right kidney is situated below the liver while the left kidney sits below the spleen and somewhat higher than its companion. The recession on the inner side of each kidney provides the opening for blood vessels, lymph glands and nerves. The ureters are the long, thin tubing allowing urine to pass from the kidneys to the bladder and also attach at these recessions.

The kidneys' primary function is to excrete wastes from protein metabolism through the urine and to regulate the body's water, electrolyte and acid-base content of the blood. These incredible organs process nearly 200 quarts of wastes and water daily. About 450 gallons of blood pass through the kidneys every day. Some of the other duties performed by the kidneys include:

- identifying the composition of the blood and knowing how and where to filter it;
- separating wastes from necessary substances in the blood; and
- controlling blood pressure and constantly overseeing the body's overall needs.

Try this beneficial kidney exercise:

Stand comfortably with feet about shoulder width apart and bend forward slightly. Rub both hands together until they feel warm. Place hands on the kidney area, right hand on right kidney, left hand on left kidney, and let the warmth from your hands penetrate the area. Rub hands up and down and in circular motions. Form a fist with your hands (thumbs inside) and gently tap the kidney area. Breathe deeply, letting the tension flow out of your body.

Do this exercise three times daily to tone and support kidney function.

Winter: Holding On and Holding In

The bladder, a thick muscular organ located in the pelvic area, serves as a reservoir for urine from the kidneys until enough is accumulated to be eliminated. The layers of muscle make it possible for the bladder to expand as it becomes full and contract when releasing. The two ureters from the kidneys enter the bladder at its back side. Their openings are covered with folds of skin acting as valves, preventing a back-flow of urine into the ureters. The bottom of the bladder narrows into the urethra which carries the urine out of the body.

A frequent occurrence many women tend to experience is urinary tract infection (UTIs), which can produce painful urination. Numerous factors contribute to these infections including:

- increased bacteria in the urethra and bladder;
- cross contamination from the rectal area;
- inflammation from injury to the urethra or bladder;
- distention of the urethra from sexual intercourse;
- pregnancy;
- kidney stones; and
- sensitivity to ingredients in bath bubbles or gels or feminine hygiene products.

Many health providers suggest drinking cranberry juice to relieve urinary tract infection symptoms. This Winter season fruit creates more acid in the urine making it a less desirable environment for bacteria. By increasing your water intake you can promote more frequent urination which helps flush bacteria from the urinary tract.

Another remedy from Nature's Pantry for UTIs is coconut oil—organic, extra virgin, fresh-pressed—due to its ability to disrupt the cellular membranes of viruses, bacteria and several other pathogens. I enjoy the flavor of coconut oil, so I just eat a teaspoonful a day as preventive nutrition. You may also enjoy adding hot water to the cranberry juice and stirring in a teaspoon of coconut oil. This warming Winter beverage supports bladder health. Please do consult your physician if symptoms persist.

Look to the seasons when choosing your cures.
~Hippocrates

Living Well in Winter

With the Winter often comes increased bouts of colds and influenza. Climate changes, fewer sunny days, breathing dry hot indoor air, drinking less water and eating a heavier diet (often lacking in fresh produce) may contribute to a lowered immune response. Preserving the health you attained in previous seasons may take extra effort in Winter, but it can be done, realistically and creatively. Let's look at two areas that can weaken our immune system: poor meal selection and lack of exercise.

First, Winter Diets can be much heavier and warmer than Spring and Summer diets. We need more protein and healthy fat for our Winter energy source. Dr. John Douillard of Boulder, Colorado's Life Spa and author of *The 3-Season Diet: Eat the Way Nature Intended* teaches that we can eat any natural food we want as long as we eat it in its season. He also encourages eating a substantial breakfast that will last until lunch, eating a larger lunch that will last until dinner, and then eating a moderate dinner that will take us to breakfast. The fast from dinner to breakfast gives your body time to repair, regenerate and release toxins. By following a sound dietary plan, especially during the Winter season, we can prevent mindless snacking and foster gradual weight loss.

If your body performs optimally on smaller, more frequent meals, be mindful in selecting a menu with a complete nutrient profile—lean protein, healthy fats, smart carbohydrates and water—to maintain your metabolic rhythms.

With overflowing platters and trays of holiday foods so attractively presented in this season, staying the course nutritiously can be difficult and sometimes discouraging. Just remember, processed carbohydrates are takers and not givers so choose your meals as wisely as you would choose a close friend. Processed, refined, pre-packaged foods deplete the body of necessary nutrients. If that isn't enough, they contribute to fatigue, obesity, respiratory weakness, lowered resistance, tooth decay, acne, decreased mental performance, PMS, and blood sugar imbalances. Take care of your inner garden by limiting these foods and balancing them with wholesome, nutritionally complete foods.

One mistake does not have to rule a person's entire life.
~Joyce Meyer, Christian author and speaker

The second way you undermine your immune system is by refusing, avoiding, or just putting off exercising. This can really backfire on you. Although you may desire to be healthy and strengthen your immune system, it seems many people think of exercise as that awful "E" word. The truth is appropriate exercise does help the body maintain balance during the Winter months. Don't use colder weather as an excuse not to exercise. Keeping a regular exercise routine all year long is essential for optimum health and wellness. Think of Winter as a time to try something new. You may consider joining a gym, a fitness group, consulting a personal trainer or just purchasing a video workout series to use in your living room. You can make all the noise you want and workout in your pjs with little or no equipment. Thankfully, there are many options that will work with your lifestyle and wellness goals.

I urge you do discover the methods that work with your unique needs. Your body is designed for movement. The more you move about outwardly, the more your inner parts move, prompting healthier circulation, respiration, muscle tone and flexibility, and digestion and elimination. Sitting in front of the fireplace with the latest novel and a cup of hot chocolate is a wonderful Winter pastime. Just don't forget to get up, stretch and move about frequently.

You must take personal responsibility. You cannot change the circumstances, the seasons, or the wind, but you can change yourself. That is something you have charge of.
~Jim Rohn, author

Winter's Wisdom

Many women I talk with tell me (much to their regret) that their lives are too full to experience the ideal, restful or regenerative aspects of Winter. Quite honestly, most of my past Winters were heavily weighted with obligations and should-do's. But I've worked on intentionally changing this.

Winter may decide to arrive in the frigid blackness of the night—with soft, quiet snow falling like a whisper—while you sleep unaware. And then when you awake, you notice another world completely different from the world you saw before you went to bed. Oh, the contrasts, but the outcome is the same. Winter has arrived. Winter is not only apparent in the physical, external world, but in your emotional, inner world as well. If you observe your life as a series of cycles (which it truly is), the latter part of your life might be considered your personal Winter. You've birthed children or careers in your youthful Springtime and nurtured both through your individual Summer season. In the Fall/Autumn of your life, with children grown and beginning their own Springtime, you reap the abundance of a successful career, healthy family and a wholesome life.

Each season has its own joyous chaos of ever-changing events, but Winter brings a certainty with it. It is here. It's cold and sometimes dark. It may be harsh or still, but it is here, no doubt about it. Winter requires attention; Winter commands respect.

Winter is the wisdom season. Truly, by the time you reach the Winter of your life, you've been-there/done-that. You have become rich in life's experiences and lessons. You have gathered and lost lifelong friends. Often you become resolute in your purpose.

Many say that older people are set in their ways. Yet I believe they've been around long enough to know what they want, when they want it and how they want it. They don't need to compromise. My life's journey has given me the honor, pleasure and blessing of knowing and loving many "Winter women." They have shared with me their joys and sorrows, pleasures and pain, wit and wisdom and some of their secrets and dreams. I desire to mature as well as these lovely wise women and pass a beautiful legacy on to the younger women in my life.

Have you thought about your own Winter season? Now is the time to plant for your abundant harvest and the inheritance in wisdom and wellness you wish to leave for the next generation of inner-garden-tenders.

25

Nature's Winter Pantry: Comfort Food for Body and Soul

Everything has seasons, and we have to be able to recognize when something's time has passed and be able to move into the next season. Everything that is alive requires pruning as well, which is a great metaphor for endings.
—Henry Cloud, clinical psychologist and author

HISTORICALLY, WINTER'S SIMPLE DIET reflected the sparseness of the season. Much of the food eaten during Winter came from the preparations made in Fall/Autumn. Home-canned fruits and vegetables lined cellar shelves ready to complement a Winter meal or snack. Root crops were prepared frequently because they stored well, provided nutrient-dense flavor and blood thickening properties, and created inner warmth during the cold weather. Perhaps you can learn from the traditions of Winters past. For a healthy Winter season, I invite you to choose from the following variety-filled list of Nature's best:

Apple

- Available year round in more than 25 varieties, often used as a dried fruit during colder months.
- The peeling has high pectin (fiber) content that helps in bowel elimination; helps lower cholesterol levels and adds moisture to bodily fluids.

Bok Choy

- Available year round, member of the cabbage family with similar nutrient values.
- High in Vitamins A and C, folate, beta-carotene, calcium and fiber.

Carrot

- Root vegetable that stores well in cool, dry, dark place.
- High in the antioxidant beta-carotene (pro-vitamin A) that protects against cancer.
- Alkaline; supports and strengthens lungs and intestines.

Cranberry

- Most commonly used for effectively treating bladder infections.
- Anti-viral and anti-bacterial components reduce activity of E.coli in the bladder and urethra.
- Freshly juiced cranberries sweetened with fresh apple, pear or grape juice is preferred over commercially prepared juices that are greatly diluted and sweetened.

Date

- Harvested from September through December, dates are high in minerals, fiber and have a laxative effect on the eliminating system.
- Provide 60-70 percent natural simple sugars, making them a good sugar substitute and a good energy producing snack or dessert during colder weather.

Grape

- Peak season from August to November; the emperor grape has long been a Thanksgiving and Christmas favorite; dried grapes—raisins—provide nutritious snacks during long winter months.

- High magnesium content promotes bowel action; supports proper kidney function; acts as effective internal cleanser for the liver; high iron content builds the blood.

Grapefruit

- Peak season is January to May, this subtropical fruit is considered an acid fruit with an alkaline reaction in the body—less acidic than a lemon.
- High in Vitamins C, B1 and B2, potassium and flavonoids; low in calories and sugar.
- Helps remove mucous congestion in the body, aids in digestion of meats, promotes healthy bowel action and when taken at bedtime, promotes sound sleep.

Kale

- Cool weather crop available in late Fall/Autumn to early Winter with peak production from December through February; member of the cabbage family.
- Flavor becomes sweeter after a light frost; high in vitamins and minerals including Vitamin A, calcium, iron, potassium and chlorophyll; provides same anti-cancer properties as other cabbage.
- One cup of kale or collard greens provides more calcium than a cup of milk.

Orange

- Available year round but most abundant from January to May, known for high Vitamin C and flavonoid content; the white pith is rich in bioflavonoids.
- Many remedies use essential oils, flowers, peel as well as pulp; high in electrolyte minerals—potassium, calcium, sodium, and magnesium.

- Helpful in respiratory disorders including asthma; strengthens the immune system; supports connective tissue and overall good health; pectin helps lower cholesterol.

Parsnip

- A Winter root vegetable that needs near freezing temperatures to fully develop its sweet nutty flavor; resembling a carrot, the root is the edible portion of the plant.
- Therapeutic value benefits the spleen, pancreas and stomach; improves bowel action by lubricating intestine; helps liver and gall bladder function; alkaline.
- Best when steamed, roasted or baked (not boiled) in their skins until tender.

Pear

- Available year round, but grow best where Summers are cool and Winters are mild.
- Sweet in flavor; wonderful digestive aid, helpful in normalizing bowel activity; provides energy during winter months.
- Healing properties help dispel excess mucous, eliminate coughing, strengthen the lungs and moisten the lungs and throat.

Pomegranate

- Native to Persia, one of the oldest fruits known to man, mentioned 30+ times in the *Holy Bible* as a greatly esteemed fruit.
- Juicy red inner seeds (pips) are rich in antioxidants that combat heart disease and some cancers.

Potato

- Cool season crop with hundreds of varieties, the russet being most well-known commercial variety; member of the nightshade family.

- Reportedly America's favorite vegetable—usually in the form of potato chips or French fries.
- Rich in potassium (higher than bananas); high fiber helps control blood sugar and blood pressure; good source of Vitamins C, B1, B2 and B3, protein and iron; complex carbohydrates provide energy.
- Potato peelings contain higher nutrient amounts than inner flesh; nearly 60 percent of potassium content is in the peelings.

Potato - Sweet

- Available year round, but in season in November and December; they are not related to the common potato.
- Offers nearly 25,000 IU of beta-carotene (Vitamin A) per serving; good source of Vitamin C, manganese, copper, Vitamin B6, potassium, iron and dietary fiber.
- Offers antioxidant protection, anti-inflammatory properties and diabetic prevention; low in calories and fat free.

Squash - Winter

- Grown in warm weather but harvested and eaten later in the season when fully matured; the hardened outer skin (rind) allows for storage through the winter.
- Includes acorn, butternut, Hubbard, pumpkin and spaghetti squash.
- Contain more natural sugars, carbohydrates and Vitamin A than summer varieties.
- Rich source of Vitamins A, C and B6, folate, potassium, magnesium, iron, calcium, and complex carbohydrates make winter squash an excellent choice for cancer protection, heart health, reproductive health and weight loss.

Tangerine

- In season from November until May with peak season in December and January.
- Shares many nutrient qualities of the orange.

Turnip

- Relative of cabbage family, usually harvested from October until March; the fall harvest produces a sweeter crop than a spring harvest.
- Root and greens are both edible, but greens provide more nutrients (Vitamin A).
- A starch food, providing only a third the calories of the same portion of a potato.
- Good source of sulfur (may be gas forming in some people), which is warming and cleansing to the body; good food choice for detoxification.
- Alkaline reaction; therapeutic benefits help with indigestion, bronchial disorders, hoarseness and diabetes.

Connie's Comments: During the Winter months, especially in colder climates, a wide variety of fresh produce may not be available, therefore, dried fruits and vegetables can provide nourishment and energy during these long cold months. Combined with beans or whole grains, hearty soups and stews will supply necessary nutrients, healthy fat and lean protein to keep the body strong, healthy and warm through the Winter season.

26

Nature's Winter Recipes: Tummy Warming for Bone-Chilling Days

There are seasons in life. Don't ever let anyone try to deny you the joy of one season because they believe you should stay in another season ... listen to yourself. Trust your instincts. Keep your perspective.
—Jane Clayson, American journalist and author

Grapefruit Juice Tonic: A Hot Drink for Cold and Flu Symptoms

1 grapefruit—preferably pink or white inner fruit (preferred to red inner fruit)
3 cups purified water
1 tsp. honey—locally grown, unfiltered

- Wash grapefruit and cut into four wedges. Use produce wash in *Nature's Spring Recipes, Chapter 11.*
- Fill 1-quart saucepan with purified water and warm over medium heat.
- Squeeze grapefruit juice from cut wedges into warming water; immerse the squeezed wedges into the water; continue simmering until hot.

- Prepare a mug with honey; pour hot grapefruit juice into mug, stir and enjoy.
- Sprinkle a pinch of cayenne powder on top, if desired.

Connie's Comments: This is an excellent drink when your body is congested. When taken before bedtime, this soothing drink promotes sound sleep. The cayenne warms the body and increases circulation which is helpful during cold and flu symptoms. If grapefruit is not available, lemon will work as well.

Note: Grapefruit interacts unfavorably (and sometimes dangerously) with many prescription medications. Please review any medications you are taking before using this grapefruit beverage.

Pomegranate Passion

1 pomegranate

- Remove seeds from pomegranate fruit by cutting the stem off and scoring the fruit end to end in 6 sections.
- Fill a large bowl with water and submerge the pomegranate while peeling away the outer skin—eliminating staining splatters. The fleshy pulp will float to the top of the water and the red seeds will sink to the bottom. Continue working all the seeds out then discard the outer peeling and pulp. Strain seeds into a storage container.
- Add the ruby-red seeds to your festive dishes for tartness, color and health benefits. They add a surprising crunch to salads, a sparkle to holiday champagne, and a tangy topper for pork and beef.

Quinoa Breakfast

Quinoa or Quinoa Flakes
Nuts, almonds or walnuts, lightly toasted and chopped
Maple syrup or raw, local honey
Milk or dairy substitute, (I use canned coconut milk)
Dried fruit, figs or currants

- Prepare quinoa (a gluten free grain) or quinoa flakes according to package directions for desired number of servings. Be sure to rinse grain (not the flakes) in a strainer before cooking, to remove protective soap-like residue.
- To cooked quinoa, add 1/2 tsp. pure maple syrup or organic honey for sweetener. Spoon cooked cereal into serving bowls. Stir in coconut milk or minimally processed cow's milk to your preferred creaminess.
- Top with chopped toasted almonds or walnuts, chopped dried figs or currants.

Connie's Comments: This breakfast provides plenty of protein, minerals and complex carbohydrates. Remember, eating a nutritiously satisfying breakfast jump-starts your metabolism with a healthy energy boost and prevents mid-morning snacking on less nutritional, empty-calorie foods that add unwanted winter weight.

Warm Red Cabbage with Bacon

Serves 4

1 small head red cabbage, shredded (about 1-pound)
2 tsp. Dijon mustard
2 tsp. red wine vinegar
3 Tbsp. olive oil
1/3 cup walnuts
3 strips bacon, crumbled in large pieces

1 tsp. freshly squeezed lemon juice
1/2 tsp. kosher salt
1/8 tsp. freshly ground black pepper
1 bunch frisee or chicory, torn into bite-size pieces (about 3 cups)

- In a large bowl, whisk together the mustard, vinegar, and 2-Tbsp. of the oil; set aside.
- In a large skillet, lightly toast the walnuts over medium heat, stirring occasionally, 5-6 minutes; remove and set aside.
- Add the bacon to skillet and cook until crispy, 3-4 minutes; remove the bacon and drain on paper towels; discard all but 1-Tbsp. of the drippings from the skillet.
- Add the remaining olive oil and the cabbage and toss to coat well; add 1/4 cup water, the lemon juice, salt and pepper and cook until soft, about 5-minutes.
- Remove from skillet and add to the vinaigrette.
- Add the frisee, walnuts and bacon crumbles; toss well.

New Year's Eve Black-Eyed-Pea Stew

Serves 10

1 pound dried black-eyed peas
1 small smoked ham hock (about 1/2 pound)
2 bay leaves
2 cloves garlic, minced
10 cups chicken broth
1/2 pound spicy Italian sausage or chorizo
1 cup white rice (not quick-cooking)
1 tsp. salt
1 cup green onion, thinly sliced
1 large red bell pepper, diced
Red pepper flakes, if desired

- In a large cooking pot, cover black-eyed peas with water to cover by 2-inches. Soak overnight. Drain well.
- In a large cooking pot, combine the drained black-eyed peas, ham hock, bay leaves, garlic and broth. Bring to a boil, reduce to a high simmer, partially cover and cook until the peas are almost tender, about 45-minutes (less cooking time if using fresh black-eyed peas).
- While above ingredients are cooking, prick the sausage skin in several places with a fork. In a medium size skillet, add about 1/8" water and sausage and bring to a boil over medium-high heat. Cook the sausage until cooked through, about 10-minutes. Set aside and discard the cooking juices. When cooled, cut the sausage into 1/4-inch slices.
- Add the sausage, rice and salt to the pot, cover again and cook until the rice is tender, about 20-minutes (less time if using pre-cooked rice). Stir in the scallions and bell pepper about 10 minutes before the rice is done. If desired, pull off any meat from the ham hock and add to the pot. Discard the bay leaves.
- Serve with warm corn bread and steamed collard greens for a comforting Southern New Year's tradition.

Connie's Comments: Fresh black-eyed peas are available in most natural foods grocers this time of year and preferable to canned. They reduce the preparation time of soaking and cooking dried black-eyed peas. I also pre-cook the rice to reduce overall cooking time of the stew. This stew can be as varied as you desire by adding stewed tomatoes, chopped kale, mustard greens or cabbage. There's such fun history behind this "good-luck" New Year's dish and you can learn more by searching Hoppin' John New Year's Recipe.

Winter White Chili

Serves 6

1 Rotisserie Chicken
1 32-ounce box organic chicken broth
2 Tbsp. olive oil
2 medium onions, diced
2 cloves garlic, minced
1 cup dry white wine
2-3 cans cannelli or great Northern beans
1/4 cup lime juice
8-oz diced green chiles or diced roasted green chiles
1 jalapeño pepper, chopped
1 Serrano pepper, chopped
1 bunch cilantro, finely snipped
1 Tbsp. oregano
1-2 Tbsp. cumin, to taste
1/4 tsp. cinnamon
1 cup jack cheese, shredded

- Pull chicken from bones, discard skin and bones, cut into bite-sized pieces.
- In crockpot on high heat, heat oil, add onion, jalapeño, Serrano and cook for 5-6 minutes; add green chilies and garlic and cook 3-5 more minutes.
- Add white wine and simmer about 5 minutes; stir well then add chicken broth and warm through.
- Add chicken, beans, oregano, cumin, and cinnamon and stir well and continue warming.
- Add lime juice and cilantro; stir; let chili mixture heat throughout.
- Add jack cheese before serving.
- Serve with warm corn bread and butter.

Connie's Comment: This is an excellent recipe for using leftover holiday turkey.

Wilted Winter Greens

Serves 2

1 Tbsp. olive oil
1 head radicchio, cored and chopped
6 kalamata olives, pitted and sliced
1-1/2 Tbsp. dried currants, cranberries, or dried cherries
1 Tbsp. oil-packed capers, drained
1/2 tsp. red pepper flakes
1 Tbsp. freshly squeezed lemon juice
1-1/2 tsp. olive oil for dressing
2 Tbsp. toasted pine nuts, walnuts, hazelnuts or pecans
1-1/2 tsp. orange zest

- Heat 1-Tbsp. olive oil in large pot or wok over medium-high heat; add endive and radicchio; cook 5-minutes stirring constantly until just wilted.
- Add olives, currants, capers, and red pepper flakes, and cook, tossing gently, 15-seconds more. Remove to serving platter.
- Drizzle greens with lemon juice and 1-1/2 tsp. olive oil; sprinkle with nuts and orange zest.

Connie's Comment: These warm winter greens are a welcome variation of the typical crisp green salad and bring a burst of flavors and textures to your Winter menu.

27

Reflections on the Season: Winter's Warming Moments

Winter is the time for comfort, for good food and warmth,
for the touch of a friendly hand, and for a talk beside the fire:
It is the time for home.
—Edith Sitwell, English poet and critic

Your Turn…

Please take a few moments to pour yourself a delicious hot drink and snuggle up in your favorite quilt while you contemplate your Winter memories and journal them here.

My favorite childhood Winter activity was:

In the Winter season I feel:

My favorite Winter foods are:

My favorite grown-up Winter activity is:

Only with winter-patience can we bring the deep desired long-awaited spring.

~Anne Morrow Lindbergh, aviation pioneer and writer, *Gift from the Sea*

28

The End of the Garden Path: Return to the Potting Shed

Each new season grows from the leftovers of the past.
That is the essence of change, and change is the essence of life.
—author unknown

The Long and Winding Garden Path

You've been on quite a journey, walking through the seasons and exercises in this almanac. Did you enjoy your stroll? I hope so. And I trust you learned as well. Now we've reached the end of the road only to begin again. The potting shed—the place where we started—has come back into sight. Let's just sit awhile to rest and reflect.

Your next seasonal journey can be quite different as you use your new tools, apply your recently acquired knowledge and listen to your inner nature. As you continue to grow with each season, the experience and wisdom you gain along the way provides a clearer *planning-and-planting* vision for the next phase of your life.

We are wonderfully designed to live harmoniously with Nature's ever changing landscape. Living fully in each season requires more than modifying our behavior according to that season. With appropriate tools we can lay the groundwork for cultivating our body's natural healing system. Eventually, you *will* reap the rewards of a strong body and strong mind.

Lessons from a Garden

TruHappiness Coach Kimberly Truitt, (KimberlyTruitt.com) invites you to "create an environment and a life that you love." She shares her wisdom on how your environment either nurtures and nourishes you or constricts and depletes you.

Today's fast-paced lifestyle tends to desensitize your internal awareness of the environment in and around you. Consequently, you would do well to develop a healthy support system for yourself. When faced with decisions about your physical, mental, emotional, and spiritual health, ask yourself the following questions:

- What do I need or want right now?
- What support do I need?
- What resources do I need? What resources are already available to me?
- What will I need to do to reach my goal?
- What will I do? When will I do it?
- Who may I ask to support my journey? (I had to learn the *art of asking* along my own wellness journey.)

This particular writing project had long been a thought, a seed, neatly tucked away in the hidden recesses of my mind until my friend and writing mentor, Judith Briles, lovingly known as The Book Shepherd, greeted me at a writing seminar, pointed her finger in my face and firmly advised me, "You need to rewrite your book!"

Well, that certainly opened a new path on my already filled road to renewal. Oh yes, it would be exciting to explore a new route. I met many wonderful writers, new friends, mentors and coaches along the way. My thinking and capabilities expanded beyond what I had previously dreamed. Small dreams grew into much grander opportunities. Careful pruning was necessary along with timing, nurturing and, of course, waiting.

Gardening experiences may progress like that. You may plant a few intentional seeds but will never truly know what the harvest will look like until harvest time.

Sometimes life becomes too large for me and comes at me too fast. Perhaps it does for you, too. As prudent and mindful women who endeavor to use appropriate tools, we can rake, weed, hoe, plow, prune and water whatever is necessary to restore our environment (internally and externally) to health, wholeness and harmony.

Nature is not a place to visit—it is home.
~Gary Snyder, American poet

Now Is the Time—Once Again

It's never too late to begin creating or re-creating your inner garden. Once you learn to actively and consistently listen to and tend your female terrain you will know how to take action before you reach a health crisis. If your internal garden grows into a severely unfavorable condition, very little energy remains for repair, recovery or restoration.

Consistent maintenance along the way takes much less time, effort and energy than waiting until later to try to regain what has been lost. I firmly believe we live in an era—economically, environmentally, politically, socially and spiritually—in which optimum wellness is critically important.

Now is a good time for you to review and update the notes you entered in your almanac. Skim your responses to the ***Your Turn*** sections of this book. Pay attention to what worked for you and what did not. Note and celebrate your progress in your journal. And remember, you are the gardener of your wellness garden. You may change, modify, discard or repeat (replant) as needed in order to reap abundant health in each future season or phase of your life.

Nature often holds up a mirror so we can see more clearly the ongoing processes of growth, renewal and transformation in our lives.
~Mary Ann Brussat, Journalist and film critic

Share the Seeds

Gardeners are some of the most generous people I know. We love to share seeds, cuttings, growing tips or the newest natural pesticide recipe. I enjoy hearing the contagious laughter of women as we swap garden stories about the biggest pumpkin or the critter that stole the prize tomato.

One of the many joys of being a woman comes from developing the art of sharing the celebration of being ourselves. With the tools, knowledge, experience and wisdom you have gained, you can not only come to celebrate every life season but to communicate your successful garden stories with other women as well. By helping others restore their inner-wellness gardens, you and I contribute to creating families, communities, and eventually a nation well-rooted in wholesome, Nature-inspired health principles and practices.

As an aging-with-vitality woman, I believe it is important to join together to share the promise, opportunity and potential of each new season. When we discover how to be well, we gain confidence in our ability, privilege and responsibility to share these seeds of wisdom with others.

Learn to be an observer in all seasons. Every single day, your garden has something new and wonderful to show you.
~unknown

Gardeners Keep Growing

The potting shed beckons. Your tools stand ready. Take a deep breath and sip a cool or warm drink depending on the calendar season you're enjoying as you read these last paragraphs. Remember, Nature never stands still and neither does your inner garden. It's always developing. Even when you're resting, much internal activity continues within you.

May you continue to use the understanding of God's seasons as a guide for your physical, emotional and spiritual well-being. Please take what you've learned during your journey through this almanac and develop into the wise and wonderful woman you long to be. I invite you to continue planting, pruning and harvesting your own unique inner garden—and pray you'll bloom beautifully, fully and well in your current season.

If you have enjoyed this journey, please thoughtfully consider sharing your experience with others by giving a helpful review of this book at *http://bit.ly/WiseWomanAlmanac-Amazon*

Have two goals: wisdom—that is, knowing and doing right—and common sense. Don't let them slip away, for they fill you with living energy, and bring you honor and respect. They keep you safe from defeat and disaster and from stumbling off the trail.

~Proverbs 3:21-23

A Garden of Information

Suggested Reading and Resource Material

If you love to laugh, don't miss some of my favorites that help lighten the way through aging:

Bolton, Martha. *Cooking with Hot Flashes*, Bethany House, 2004.
Swartz, Susan. *Juicy Tomatoes: Plain Truths, Dumb Lies and Sisterly Advice About Life After 50*, New Harbinger Publications, 2000.
Walker, Laura Jensen. *Mentalpause: And Other Midlife Laughs*, Revell (Baker Publishing Group), 2001.

We all want healthy food that tastes good and heals at the same time. Some of my favorite resources include:

Cordain, Ph.D., Loren. *The Paleo Diet*, John Wiley & Sons, Inc., 2002.
Douillard, John. *The 3-Season Diet*, Three River Press, 2000.
Goulart, Frances Sheridan. *Super Healing Foods*, Parker Publishing Company, 1995.
Haas, M.D., Elson M. *Staying Healthy with the Seasons*, CelestialArts, 1981.
Jensen, D.C., Bernard. *Foods That Heal: A Guide to Understanding and Using the Healing Powers of Natural Foods*, Avery (Penguin Putnam, Inc.), 1993.
Murray, N.D., Michael T. *The Healing Power of Foods: Nutrition Secrets for Vibrant Health and Longevity*, Prima Publishing, 1993.
Murray, N.D., Michael T. *The Healing Power of Herbs*, Prima Publishing, 1995.
Pitchford, Paul. *Healing with Whole Foods*, North Atlantic Books, 1993.
Pollan, Michael. *In Defense of Food*, The Penguin Press, 2008.

For general health and well-being information focusing on the interconnectedness of our bodies and Nature, these are a few of my go-to resources:

Cherniske, Stephen and Kather, M.D., Natalie. *The Metabolic Makeover*, Altea Media, LLC, 2014.

Jensen, D.C., Bernard. *Empty Harvest*, Avery (Penguin Putnam Inc.), 1995.

Monte, Tom. *World Medicine: The East West Guide to Healing Your Body*, G.P. Putnam's Sons, 1993.

Northrup, M.D., Christiane. *The Wisdom of Menopause: Creating Physical and Emotional Health During the Change*, Bantam Books (The Random House Publishing Group), 2012.

Northrup, M.D., Christiane. *Women's Bodies, Women's Wisdom*, Bantam Books, 2010.

And for my scriptural references I search a variety of translations from the *Holy Bible* including:

The Living Bible
The New International Version
The New Living Translation
Peterson, Eugene H. *The Message*, NavPress, 2014.

Some of my favorite websites include:

DrAxe.com – Health, Fitness, Natural Remedies

DrWeil.com – The Anti-Inflammatory Food Pyramid

LifeSpa.com – Dr. John Douillard's 3-Season Plan

TheMetabolicMakeover.com – The simple science of creating energy with nutrition

WHFoods.com – Food nutrient values – identifies the world's healthiest foods

WellnessForAllSeasons.com – Sign up for my blog to get the latest recipes and tips.

Appreciations

Community effort can produce an abundant yield in the field or garden. Similarly, community effort helped bring this book to fruition. Many dear friends, clients, colleagues and family encouraged, instructed, edited, scolded and prayed me through this writing season, and I am grateful.

A heartfelt thanks to my amazing daughters, Jennifer and Kaci, for always believing in me and encouraging me to follow my passion; to my husband, Willie, for reminding me to stay the course; to my parents, who in their late-80s, are still living life "being" well; to my sister, Carol, who shared in the chores and the fun that make up our sister memories; and to my precious granddaughters, Kelln and Quinn, who are showing me the delight of the grandmothering season!

I appreciate and admire the creative talents of Nick Zelinger (*NZgraphics.com*) for his cover design and book layout; Micah Billingsley (*ThriceCreative.com*), for the seasonal tree illustrations; Kaci Head for the Potting Shed photograph and Stephanie Monaghan for the female anatomy illustration. Their artistry brought vibrant life to this book.

A bushel of thanks to Kelly Johnson of Cornerstone Virtual Assistance (*CornerstoneVA.com*) and Judith Briles, The Book Shepherd (*TheBookShepherd.com*), for editing, proofreading, formatting, and giving authoring advice.

A heartfelt thanks to many older, wiser "mother-mentor-friends" who kept me moving forward and taught me how to age with vitality, because each season truly is a new beginning. Each of you brought blessings to my journey. Thank you.

About the Author ...
Meet Connie Pshigoda

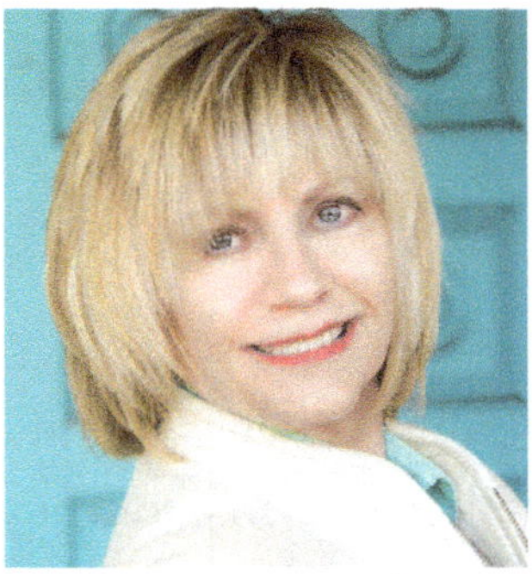

The phrase "living well" will take on a whole new meaning once you read Connie's writings. Her passion for optimum health and her love for her Creator and His Creation, have brought her to this season of her life—this part of her journey.

Connie Pshigoda is a Certified Nutritional Therapist, Natural Health Coach, founder of Wellness For All Seasons and published author. She brings her passion for Nature's nourishment "to the table" in her writings, coaching and presentations. Her 40+ year education and career journey in holistic health has convinced her that the time-tested truths of choosing from Nature's pantry, rather than the manufactured man-made foods, promises a life of exceptional health and vitality!

Her total wellness approach draws on the wisdom of Nature's seasons to improve overall health and well-being using the healing properties and preventive nutrition of Nature's plant foods. Using this wisdom, Connie shows you how to manage your menus with a seasonal flavor and flair. She guides her readers and clients through a wellness process of rebuilding, restoring, renewing so that they may reap the rewards of a vibrant life—in every season. Her blog, *Garden Gatherings*, is rich with seasonal advice and delicious recipes.

Growing up on a farm provided the foundation that seeded and fertilized her wellness career. She now enjoys the great outdoors of Colorado with her husband, two daughters and their families.

How to Work with Connie

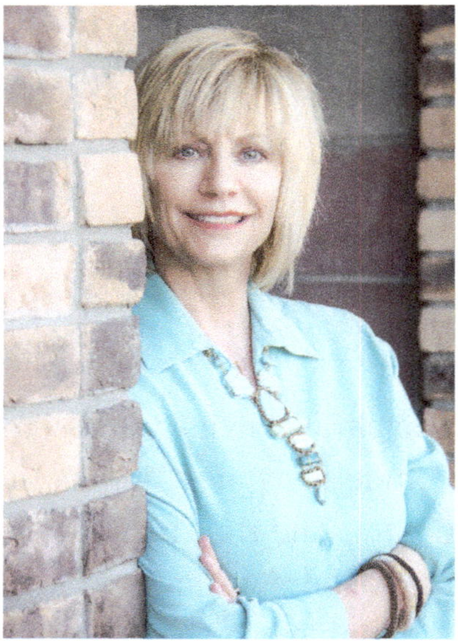

Connie's lively and informative approach takes you on a journey through Spring, Summer, fall and Winter. her farming experience lends wit, practicality and wisdom as she guides you through planting, nourishing and reaping abundant health in your body's inner garden.

For Speaking ... you will come away from her presentations with:

- A **clear understanding** of nutritional and healing properties of plant foods.
- An **increased awareness** of environmental influences on your health.
- **Simple strategies and natural solutions** for improving health

Connie's dynamic and informative coaching style provides insightful recommendations for your personal health questions and concerns.

For Coaching ... she coaches one-on-one or to small groups, providing wellness tools that change participants' attention to nature's seasons and foods and the effect on their health-style. her mindful menus bring vitality to your table as well as your body.

Follow Connie on social media and contact her through her website or email for her availability to speak to your group or to engage her for personal coaching:

Connie@WellnessForAllSeasons.com

WellnessForAllSeasons.com

Wellness4AllSeasons **ConniePshigoda**

Wellness Coaching is a professional service that provides information, insight, feedback and guidance to assist you in changing your current unhealthy habits and behavior to bring about your desired wellness goals. Connie partners with you to assess your health challenges or desires and helps you design a personalized plan of action to meet your needs. This coach/client collaboration creates a powerful partnership that allows you to:

- Do more than you might on your own
- Create momentum and consistency
- Take more effective & focused actions
- Enjoy the journey while improving your health and well-being

"Connie helped me understand the importance and benefit of using a plant based diet and supplements to naturally regulate my blood sugar imbalances. In the past ten months of following Connie's nutritional plan, my energy levels have stabilized so now I no longer experience the "highs and lows" throughout the day. Even my physician was pleased to see my healthier lab reports. I'm experiencing better overall health as well as noticing a decrease in the bouts of respiratory issues."

—Joan M., Colorado

People hire a wellness life coach when they want to . . .

- Improve health, reduce stress and create balance in life
- Stop that "out-of-control" feeling with family, work & other daily factors
- Achieve personal optimum wellness
- Reduce stress and illness
- Slow aging and increase energy levels
- Stop experiencing seasonal "sick-days"
- Jump start commitment to a lifelong wellness plan

NOTES

NOTES

NOTES